Virology Division

DIAGNOSTIC VIROLOGY

Illustrated by Light and Electron Microscopy

THIRD EDITION

G. D. Hsiung

IN COLLABORATION WITH
CAROLINE K. Y. FONG

YALE UNIVERSITY PRESS
NEW HAVEN AND LONDON

Designed by Sally Harris
and set in Times Roman type.
Printed in the United States of America by
The Murray Printing Co., Westford, Mass.

Library of Congress Cataloging in Publication Data

Hsiung, G. D. (Gueh Djen), 1918–
    Diagnostic virology.
    Includes index.
    1. Viruses—Identification—Handbooks, manuals, etc.
2. Virus diseases—Diagnosis—Handbooks, manuals, etc.
3. Microscopy, Medical—Handbooks, manuals, etc.
I. Fong, Caroline K. Y.   II. Title.   [DNLM: 1. Virus
diseases—Diagnosis—Laboratory manuals.   2. Virology—
Laboratory manuals.   QW 25 H873d]
QR387.H74   1982   616'.0194   82–4835
ISBN 0–300–02888–1   AACR2

10 9 8 7 6 5 4 3 2 1

This edition is dedicated
to the memory of
ROBERT HOLT GREEN, M.D.
(1911–1981)

Dr. Green, a physician, a researcher, a teacher, and a friend,
first opened the author's eyes to the gaps in knowledge
between clinical medicine and basic research in virology.

Contents

Part 3. Recognition and Characterization of Viruses by Virus Morphology and Virus-Induced Cellular Changes

RNA VIRUSES

DNA VIRUSES

Part 4. Cell Culture

Illustrations

Tables

Preface to the Third Edition

The first edition of this book, published as a laboratory manual in 1964, was intended to be used by students enrolled in postgraduate courses in diagnostic virology. In the ensuing years, it has been used in laboratories as a handbook for virus recognition and characterization, as a teaching guide in classrooms for medical students, and as a laboratory manual in our own postgraduate course in diagnostic and experimental virology. In order to illustrate some of the characteristics of virus-induced cellular changes in cultures, the book contained many photographs taken under light microscopy. Despite the rapid growth in the field of technical procedures in diagnostic virology, the photographs and illustrations are still indispensable. Of particular interest, however, in the present edition is the addition of electron micrographs of virus morphology in negatively stained preparations and in infected cells.

Considerable revision of many chapters has been undertaken in order to make the information current. Due to the breakthroughs in knowledge of hepatitis viruses and rotaviruses and to the isolation and propagation of human papovavirus in culture, several new chapters, including illustrative electron micrographs, have been added.

This handbook is now designed primarily as a visual aid for the recognition of virus-induced cellular changes and virus morphology, especially of those agents encountered in human diseases. It is intended to assist those individuals involved in clinical laboratory work, as well as physicians and teachers, in recognizing viruses and virus-induced cellular changes. The descriptive information serves as a guide to the illustrative materials. In-depth discussions on theories and mechanisms of virus replication and descriptions of procedures for virus isolation and identification are limited in order to maintain the ease of use that a handbook demands.

The book is divided into four parts. Part 1 deals with general principles of diagnostic virology and provides guidelines for collecting specimens. Part 2 describes the essential techniques that are most commonly used in a virology laboratory for virus isolation and identification and for antibody determination; it is arranged in nine chapters and can be adapted as a teaching guide or schedule for a course in medical virology. Part 3 comprises the major portion of the book. It is subdivided into virus groups representing those agents that may be encountered in a clinical virology laboratory; it lists the various virus types and gives a brief description of the general properties of each group. Distinct characteristics of each virus type are illustrated by photographs, either macroscopic or microscopic, of virus-induced changes or, through electron microscopy, of virus particles or virus-infected cells. The final part, part 4, deals with procedures for the preparation of primate and nonprimate tissue cells in culture and describes the common endogenous virus contaminants; it emphasizes the simian virus group, of which the tissue culture virologist should be particularly aware.

The photographs in this book may be readily applied to viruses infecting members of the animal kingdom other than human beings, and the procedures described herein may be useful to those engaged in research on viruses of animal as well as of human origin. All measurements of photographs are final magnifications (approximately).

The text contains no references, but a short list of review papers and selected specific articles are provided at the end of parts 1, 2, and 4 and at the end of each chapter in part 3 as supplementary readings.

ACKNOWLEDGMENTS

The authors are grateful to Kari Hastings for her devotion in editing the entire book. Without her continuing efforts in collecting and assembling the materials presented in the new chapters, it would have been impossible to complete this book in time for publication.

Our thanks also go to Dr. Frank Michalski, director of the Clinical Virology Laboratory, St. Michael's Medical Center, Newark, New Jersey, for reviewing the entire manuscript. We also wish to thank Mary Wright for her patience in typing and retyping the manuscript and Barbara Nunes for preparing the photographs and illustrations.

Special thanks are due to Dr. N. Karabatsos for his contribution of the togaviridae chapter, to Dr. J. Bove for his review of the hepatitis chapter, and to Drs. W. Henle, M. August, F. Bia, S. Klaus, and J. Wright for the contribution of their unpublished light and electron micrographs; permissions granted by publishers for the reproduction of photographs are also acknowledged. Suggestions made by participants in our post-graduate course and in a training program supported by a Clinical Virology Training grant from the National Institutes of Health and held at the Virology Laboratory, West Haven Veterans Administration Medical Center, were invaluable.

Abbreviations

General

ALF	allantoic fluid
AMF	amniotic fluid
AO	acridine orange staining
CAM	chorioallantoic membrane
CNS	central nervous system
CPE	cytopathic effect
CSF	cerebrospinal fluid
DNA	deoxyribonucleic acid
EM	electron microscopy
HAd	hemadsorption
H&E	hematoxylin-eosin staining
PFU	plaque-forming unit
RBC	red blood cells
RDE	receptor-destroying enzyme
RNA	ribonucleic acid
TC	tissue culture
$TCID_{50}$	tissue culture infectious dose, 50% end point
URI	upper-respiratory illness
UV	ultraviolet

Cell cultures

A549	cell line derived from human lung carcinoma
BEK	bovine embryonic kidney
BHK-21	cell line derived from baby hamster kidney tissue
BSC-1	cell line derived from African green monkey kidney tissue
CE	chicken embryo fibroblast
GMK	green monkey kidney
GPE	guinea pig embryo
HAM	human amnion cell
HDF	human diploid fibroblast
HEK	human embryonic kidney
HeLa	cell line derived from carcinoma of human cervix
Hep-2	cell line derived from epidermoid carcinoma of human larynx
HLF	human embryonic lung fibroblast
KB	cell line derived from carcinoma of human nasopharynx
MK	monkey kidney
patas MK	patas monkey kidney
RhMK	rhesus monkey kidney
RK	rabbit kidney
Vero	cell line derived from African green monkey kidney tissue

Viruses and diseases

AAV	adeno-associated virus
BL	Burkitt's lymphoma
BKV	a human papovavirus
CMV	cytomegalovirus
EBV	Epstein-Barr virus
ECHO	enteric cytopathogenic human orphan virus
EEE	Eastern equine encephalitis virus

HSV-1	herpes simplex virus type 1	IEM	immunoelectron microscopy
HSV-2	herpes simplex virus type 2	IF	immunofluorescent
JCV	a human papovavirus	IgG	immunoglobulin G
LCM	lymphocytic choriomeningitis virus	IgM	immunoglobulin M
		IP	immunoperoxidase
MINIA	monkey intranuclear inclusion agent	NT	neutralization
		RIA	radioimmunoassay
NDV	Newcastle disease virus		
NPC	nasopharyngeal carcinoma		
PML	progressive multifocal leuko-encephalopathy	*Media and solutions*	
RSV	respiratory syncytial virus	BME	basal medium, Eagle's
SA	simian agent	BSA	bovine serum albumin
SSPE	subacute sclerosing panen-cephalitis	BSS	balanced salt solution
		CS	calf serum
SV	simian virus	EDTA	ethylene diaminetetraacetic acid
SV_5	simian virus 5 (a parain-fluenza virus)	EES	Eagle's basal medium pre-pared with Earle's BSS
SV_{40}	simian virus 40 (vacuolating virus of monkey)	EHS	Eagle's basal medium pre-pared with Hanks' BSS
URI	upper-respiratory illness	ELS	Earle's BSS with lactalbu-min hydrolysate plus se-rum, Melnick medium B
VSV	vesicular stomatitis virus		
VZV	varicella-zoster virus		
WEE	Western equine encephalitis virus	ES	Earle's medium special for myxovirus
		FBS	fetal bovine serum
Serologic tests		HK	human kidney growth me-dium, Hsiung
CF	complement-fixation		
ELISA	enzyme-linked immunosor-bent assay	HLS	Hanks' BSS with lactalbumin hydrolysate plus serum, Melnick medium A
HA	hemagglutinin or hemaggluti-nation	MEM	minimum essential medium
HAd	hemadsorption	PBS	phosphate-buffered saline
HAd-I	hemadsorption-inhibition	PTA	phosphotungstate acid
HI	hemagglutination-inhibition	VB	Veronal buffer solution

PART 1: General Aspects

1. General Principles and Recent Developments in Diagnostic Virology

Although extensive progress has been made in recent years in molecular virology, the laboratory diagnosis of viral disease is still not widely practiced. Viral diagnostic facilities generally are available only in conjunction with research laboratories and state health departments and are rarely operated within a clinical microbiology setting. To a large extent, this situation is a reflection of the stringent procedures and specialized knowledge necessary for conducting virological tests. The average health professional remains unfamiliar with viral diagnostic procedures, including that for the proper collection of specimens for viral culture. However, with the development of rapid and sensitive techniques for detecting viral antigens and the development of effective drugs for the treatment of some viral diseases, the attitudes of physicians toward diagnostic virology have changed considerably in recent years.

CURRENT CONCEPTS IN VIRAL DIAGNOSIS

Frequently, when a physician is unable to make a specific diagnosis of a patient's febrile illness, he or she may comment that the patient "probably has a virus." All too often, however, identification of which one of the many viruses that may be causing the patient's illness does not seem important to the attending physician because specific therapy usually is not available.

Today, chemotherapy treatment of herpes encephalitis is possible, although evidence of herpes simplex virus infection by brain biopsy usually is sought prior to instituting therapy. Similarly, when herpes simplex virus is isolated from the genital tract of a pregnant woman near term, a caeserian section is recommended in order to avoid neonatal infection. In both instances, specific viral diagnosis is desirable. Thus, the diagnostic virologist is charged with the responsibility of identifying viruses in clinical specimens as accurately and as quickly as possible in order to meet the need for the proper management of such patients.

The ensuing chapters describe the use of selected cell-culture systems in combination with light and electron microscopy as a means of recognizing and characterizing viruses and virus-induced cellular changes. Chapters on each major virus group are designed specifically to provide guidelines for rapid diagnosis of viral infection, with special reference to some of the unusual situations, such as mixed viral infections, that may be encountered.

RECENT DEVELOPMENTS IN IMMUNOLOGIC TECHNIQUES

Many serological tests are currently in use for the diagnosis of viral diseases; complement-fixation, hemagglutination-inhibition, and neutralization tests are commonly used. In recent years, the sensitivity of serologic tests has been enhanced by the use of specific viral antibody labeled with markers in, for example, immunofluorescent staining (IF), enzyme-linked immunosorbent assay (ELISA), or radioimmunoassay (RIA). These newer immunologic tests, especially ELISA, are of particular value for detecting those viral agents that are not cultivable in cell culture or those viruses with a slow growth rate in culture. In these instances, diagnosis of viral disease is almost totally dependent upon immunologic tests. These tests have also been extremely helpful in epidemiological studies. However, because antigenic crossing often occurs and highly specific reagents may be lacking, accurate diagnosis frequently cannot be assured until the agent is isolated and characterized.

THE USE OF ELECTRON MICROSCOPY FOR ACCURATE AND RAPID DIAGNOSIS

Direct visualization of virus particles under an electron microscope is one of the most reliable methods for recognizing a specific virus. Differentiation of poxvirus from herpesvirus in skin lesion by electron microscopy (EM) has been used for several decades. The recognition of Epstein-Barr herpesvirus in cultured lymphoblastic cells, of papovavirus particles in the brain cells of patients with progressive multifocal leukoencephalopathy (PML), and of measles virus nucleocapsids in the brain cells of those with subacute sclerosing panencephalitis (SSPE) are examples of diagnoses of human viral diseases made possible by EM. The discovery of two kinds of particles, surface antigen and Dane particles, in the sera of patients with hepatitis B and of small virus particles in stool samples of hepatitis A patients was made possible by EM. Furthermore, the development of immunoelectron microscopy (IEM) has advanced rapidly in recent years and provides a more useful and sensitive refinement than simple electron microscopic examination. Identification of the Norwalk agent in stool samples of patients with nonbacterial gastroenteritis and recognition of the rotavirus in stool samples of children with infantile diarrhea would have been missed had not EM or IEM techniques been applied.

In the past, the tedious and time-consuming procedures associated with the preparation of specimens for EM examination have hindered considerably its application in the clinical laboratory. However, in recent years improved technology has simplified many of the procedures and reduced the time necessary for specimen preparation, bringing electron microscopy within the scope of a clinical virology laboratory.

GROWTH OF INTEREST IN VIRUS GROUPS

The development of new techniques has greatly influenced the growth of interest in certain groups of viruses. The waves of interest, the surges of research activity, and the demands of viral diagnosis fluctuate from year to year, as represented by the number of publications reported in *Index Medicus* (figure 1). Apparently because of the successful use of live poliovirus vaccine in the early

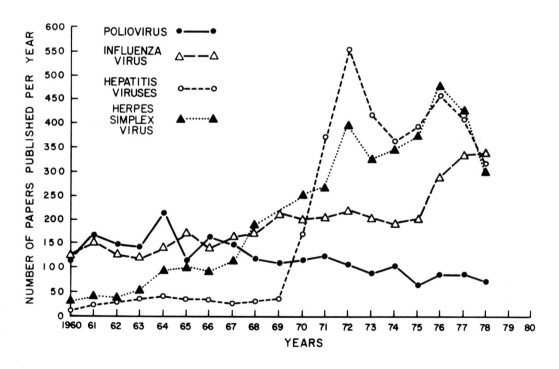

Figure 1. Number of publications concerning four representative groups of viruses reported annually in the *Index Medicus*, 1960–1978 (from G. D. Hsiung, *Yale J. Biol. Med.* 53: 1, 1980).

1960s in reducing the incidence of poliomyelitis, interest in the study of polio-viruses has gradually declined. On the other hand, influenza virus infections occur annually in sporadic or epidemic form, creating a constant public concern; therefore, the steady interest in this virus over the years is understandable. The threat of a possible pandemic of swine influenza in 1975–1976 probably accounts for the increase in the number of papers on influenza published in that year and the two following years.

Although viral hepatitis has long been recognized as an important clinical entity, until recently the number of papers published on hepatitis was small. The discovery of hepatitis B antigens in patients' sera, the recognition of viral particles by EM, and the application of radioimmunoassay and other immuno-logic methods for detecting hepatitis B virus antigens and antibody doubtless were responsible for the increased interest in hepatitis B. In addition, recogni-tion of the agent of hepatitis A, made possible by the use of EM and IEM, was followed by more papers devoted to this subject.

Very few studies of herpesviruses, including herpes simplex virus, were pub-lished in the early 1960s, perhaps because these agents were not considered to be causes of major human disease, other than the occasional cases of herpes encephalitis. Great interest in the herpesviruses, however, has been stimulated by the epidemiological association between herpes simplex virus type 2 and cervical cancer; the link between Epstein-Barr herpesvirus and Burkitt's lym-phoma, nasopharyngeal carcinoma, and infectious mononucleosis; the increasing rate of cytomegalovirus isolations from renal transplant recipients and of vari-cella-zoster virus from patients treated with immunosuppressive drugs; the successful treatment of herpes simplex encephalitis by adenine arabinoside; and the recognition of herpesvirus as an important cause of sexually transmitted disease.

SUMMARY

The expansion and growth of interest in diagnostic virology is no doubt partly due to advances in technology. Recent developments in tissue transplantation, cancer chemotherapy, and the development of antiviral therapy have greatly augmented the need for rapid and accurate diagnosis of viral infections. Virolo-gists are no longer dependent upon laboratory animals and cell cultures to iso-late and identify viruses; they now may also use alternative methods, including electron microscopy and immunoelectron microscopy as well as recently de-veloped immunologic tests. If chemotherapy of more viral diseases becomes a reality, the need for specific and rapid diagnosis of viral disease will become even more pressing. Thus, a diagnostic virology laboratory may soon offer services similar to those provided by a diagnostic bacteriology laboratory and thereby become an important branch of clinical medicine.

2. Collecting and Handling Specimens for Virological Studies

COLLECTION OF SPECIMENS

Successful isolation of viruses from clinical material depends largely on the proper collection and handling of specimens. Ideally, specimens for virus studies should be collected in sterile containers and as early as possible in the course of the disease (figure 2) or on the date of admission if the patient is hospitalized. The appropriate specimens should be delivered promptly to the virology laboratory. All samples should be properly labeled and accompanied by such information as the patient's name, age, sex, date of onset of illness, and presumptive clinical diagnosis; the latter is essential for selection of the most sensitive test system. A summary of the types of specimens to be collected from patients suspected of having viral infection is listed in table 1.

Throat washings. These can be obtained by having the patient gargle several times with 5 to 10 ml of normal saline; usually 0.5% gelatin or bovine albumin is added to protect the unstable viruses.

Throat, nasopharyngeal, or rectal swabs. Swabs are placed in tubes containing 2 ml of Hanks' balanced salt solution (BSS) with a protein stabilizer, 0.5% gelatin or calf serum, or directly into culture tubes with double the usual concentration of antibiotics. Virocult® (from Virocult® Medical Wire & Equipment Co., Cleveland, Ohio) or any similarly prepared swabs may be used.

Stool specimens. Stools (5 to 10 gm) are preferable to rectal swabs since at any given time only a small amount of virus may be present in fecal material.

Cerebrospinal fluid (CSF), pleural or pericardial effusions. Several milliliters of each (ideally 5 to 10 ml) are collected in a sterile tube.

Urine. Freshly voided urine, preferably the first morning specimen (10 to 50 ml), are collected in a sterile bottle.

Blood samples. Blood should be drawn from all patients. The first sample (10 to 15 ml of clotted blood) should be collected on admission and a second specimen 2 to 3 weeks later, or before discharging the patient. Occasionally

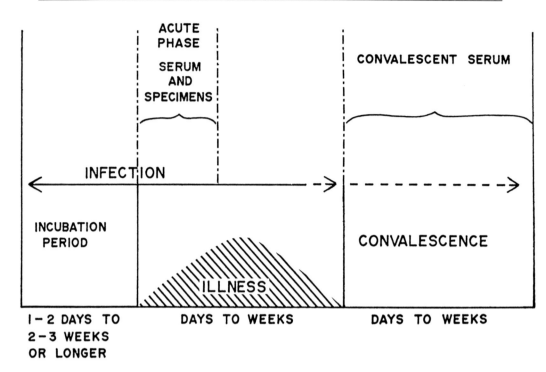

Figure 2. Time schedule for collecting specimens for virus studies (from G. D. Hsiung and R. H. Green, *Virology and Rickettsiology,* vol. 1, pt. 1, p. 4).

Table 1. Specimens to Be Collected from Patients Suspected of Viral Infection

Virus Suspected	Clinical Disease Commonly Associated with Virus	Clinical Specimens[a]	Postmortem Materials
Enterovirus	aseptic meningitis, pleurodynia, myocarditis, pericarditis, herpangina, poliomyelitis	stool, rectal swab, throat swab, CSF	spinal cord & other CNS tissues, blood, pericardial fluid, tissues with pathological lesions, colon contents
Rhinovirus	nonspecific febrile illness, common cold, afebrile URI	nasal washings, nasopharyngeal swabs	repiratory tract, lungs
Togavirus	acute febrile illness, encephalitis, aseptic meningitis	blood	brain & CNS tissues, blood

Virus Suspected	Clinical Disease Commonly Associated with Virus	Clinical Specimens[a]	Postmortem Materials
Influenza and parainfluenza viruses	pharyngitis, croup, bronchiolitis, pneumonia, URI	nasopharyngeal washing, nasal swab, throat swab, blood, gargle washing, urine	lung, trachea, blood
Mumps virus	parotitis, orchitis, aseptic meningitis	throat swab, blood, urine	
Measles virus	measles, SSPE, encephalitis	throat swab, blood, urine	blood, CNS tissues, lung
Respiratory syncytial virus	croup, bronchiolitis, pneumonia	throat swab, nasal swab	lung, trachea
Reovirus	respiratory illness (?), diarrhea (?)	throat swab, rectal swab	feces, blood, lung
Rotavirus	gastroenteritis	stool	intestine & colon contents
Rubella virus	congenital rubella rash, lymphadenopathy	throat swab, rectal swab, urine	placental & fetal tissues
Adenovirus	acute respiratory disease, pneumonia, pharyngoconjunctival fever, keratoconjunctivitis, etc.	throat swab, rectal swab, stool, eye swab	lung, colon contents
Herpes simplex virus	gingivostomatitis, keratoconjunctivitis, herpes labialis, genital herpes, encephalitis	vesicle fluid, throat swab or mouth washing, vaginal swab, brain biopsy	brain tissues with lesions, other organs
Varicella-zoster virus	chicken pox, herpes zoster	vesicle fluid, lesion swab	
Cytomegalovirus	mononucleosis, hepatitis, pneumonia, cytomegalo-inclusion disease	buffy coat, urine, throat swab	lung, kidney, salivary gland
Poxvirus	eczema vaccinatum, smallpox	local lesion fluid, pus, crust, blood	liver, spleen, blood
Hepatitis virus	jaundice	serum, stool, liver, kidney	liver, blood, colon contents

[a] For antibody determinations, acute-phase serum should be collected immediately after onset; convalescent serum should be collected 2 to 4 weeks after onset.

citrated or heparinized blood is required in order to separate blood cell populations.

Autopsy materials. These should be obtained as soon as possible after death; collect aseptically and do *not* use preservatives. For each organ removed, separate instruments and individual containers should be used.

STORAGE AND TRANSPORTATION OF SPECIMENS

Since most viruses are unstable, specimens for virus isolation should be kept cool. Speed in delivering specimens to the laboratory is of great importance, and refrigeration is necessary if delays are unavoidable. If possible, specimens should be processed and inoculated immediately upon arrival at the laboratory; if there is a short delay, for example of a few hours, refrigerate at 4°C. For longer periods of storage freeze samples, preferably at −70°C but *not* at −20°C.

If specimens are shipped by mail they should be packed with dry ice in sealed containers.

PROCESSING SPECIMENS FOR VIRUS ISOLATION

Blood specimens. Blood should *not* be frozen. Centrifuge soon after the clot has formed to obtain the serum. Serum should be separated from the clotted blood as soon as possible and kept frozen, preferably at −70°C. In certain instances, heparinized or citrated whole blood or buffy coat containing leukocytes may be used for virus isolation attempts.

Body fluids (including cerebrospinal fluid, pleural fluid, vesicle fluid, and urine). Inoculate directly into test cultures.

Throat swabs, eye swabs, nose swabs, etc. Place directly into test culture, with double concentrations of antibiotics,* or inoculate collection/transport fluids into test culture.

Stools. Process as follows:

1. Make a 20% suspension of stool by adding 4 gm stool to 16 ml Hanks' BSS.
2. Shake vigorously for 30 minutes in stoppered flask containing glass beads if available.
3. Centrifuge at 3000 rpm for 30 minutes, preferably in refrigerated centrifuge.
4. Remove and recentrifuge supernatant at 3000 rpm for 30 minutes.
5. Filter through a 450-nm millipore membrane and add antibiotics to final concentration of: penicillin, 500 units per ml; streptomycin, 500 μg per ml; neomycin, 100 μg per ml; amphotericin B, 2.5 μg per ml; or gentamicin, 100 μg per ml.
6. Inoculate into suitable culture system.

*Preference of antibiotic solution varies among laboratories. For additional information, see p. 270.

Autopsy materials (including spinal cord, lung, etc.). Process as follows:

1. Grind autopsy tissues with either a mortar and pestle or a homogenizer.
2. Add 1–2 ml Hanks' BSS and grind until smooth; add an additional 1–2 ml BSS, grind, and gradually add BSS until a 10%–20% suspension is obtained.
3. Add antibiotics as stated above.
4. Centrifuge at 1000 rpm for 15 minutes, inoculate supernatant and cell pellet into appropriate culture system.
5. For isolation of cell-associated viruses, mince or trypsinize tissues to avoid cell lysis (see part 4).
6. Cell suspensions of minced or trypsinized tissue should be diluted to a 10% concentration with growth medium. Cultivate in culture flask or co-cultivate with susceptible cell cultures.

SEROLOGIC TESTS

Serologic tests are necessary when virus isolation is impracticable and to determine the significance of the isolation of certain viruses. When serologic tests are uscd for diagnosis, paired sera are required, one obtained in the acute stage of the illness and another 10 to 21 or more days after onset. Occasionally, single serum taken shortly after illness can be used for antibody detection in the IgM fraction, although the rheumatoid factor must be controlled. The procedures for various serologic tests are described in part 2.

For more detailed procedures on specimen collection and handling, virus isolation, and serologic tests, the references listed on page 13 are recommended. Additional information can be found in the various manuals and textbooks.

SAFETY PRECAUTIONS

Safety Precautions for Personnel Working in a Virology Laboratory

All personnel working with infectious agents or handling materials suspected of haboring pathogens are exposed to the risk of infection. Therefore proper safety precautions and careful basic laboratory regulations as described below must be followed. These precautions are particularly critical in a virology laboratory where viral contaminants are a constant source of concern, even in the uninoculated "normal" control cultures. It is advisable to have serum samples taken from all personnel working in a virology laboratory before they start to work, and thereafter once a year, and stored in a freezer for later tests.

Specific Laboratory Safety Rules

1. Keep all vials, culture tubes, flasks, etc., containing virus *tightly stoppered* when not being used.

2. Do not mouth pipette; all dilutions and inoculations of virus are to be done with pipetting devices. Discard contaminated pipettes into containers with disinfectant.

3. *Never* put a contaminated pipette on the surface of your workbench. *Never* walk around with a contaminated pipette in your hand. *Never* discard any virus-containing fluids in the sink.

4. No eating, drinking, or smoking in the laboratory and no storage of food or beverages in laboratory cabinets or refrigerators is allowed.

5. Wash hands thoroughly before leaving the laboratory. (Remove surgical gloves before leaving work area.)

6. Scrub down the bench tops with disinfectant at the end of each day.

7. Wear lab coats at all times when working in a virology laboratory.

General Laboratory Safety Procedures

1. All contaminated materials, including contaminated pipettes, needles, and syringes, should be properly labeled and autoclaved before being washed or disposed of. No infectious substances should be allowed to enter the building drainage system.

2. Stock solutions of suitable disinfectants, including 10% formalin and/or 70% ethanol, should be available at the work site.

3. Special attention should be given to personnel in contact with infected animals. Water bottles or cages in which infected animals are kept should be sterilized after use. Care must be taken to discard infected animal carcasses and tissues that are sent to the incinerator for disposal. Infected embryonic eggs should be treated in the same manner.

In summary. Autoclave or steam heat, when it can be applied, is the most effective means of sterilization. Where autoclave cannot be applied, ultraviolet light is effective in decontaminating air and surfaces. In addition, immunization of personnel should be carried out wherever vaccines are available for use against particular viruses being handled in the laboratory.

SUPPLEMENTARY READING FOR PART 1

Books

Andrewes, C. H., Pereira, H. G., and Wildy, P. *Viruses of vertebrates.* 4th ed. London: Bailliere, Tindall and Cassell, 1978.

Dulbecco, R., and Ginsberg, H. S. *Virology.* 3rd ed. Harperstown, Md.: Harper & Row, Inc., 1980.

Fenner, F. O., and White, D. O. *Medical virology.* 3rd ed. New York: Academic Press, 1976.

Hsiung, G. D., ed. Recent advances in clinical virology. New York: Praeger, 1980.

Hsiung, G. D., and Green, R. H., eds. *Virology and rickettsiology,* vol. 1, pts. 1 and 2. Handbook series in clinical laboratory science, Section H. West Palm Beach, Fla.: CRC Press, 1978.

Kurstak, E., and Kurstak, C., eds. *Comparative diagnosis of viral diseases*, vol. 1 and 2. New York: Academic Press, 1977.

Lennette, E. H., Balows, A., Hausler, W. J., Jr., and Truant, J. P., eds. *Manual of clinical microbiology*. 3rd ed. Washington, D. C.: American Society for Microbiology, 1980.

Lennette, E. H., and Schmidt, N. J., eds. *Diagnostic procedures for viral, rickettsial and chlamydial infections*. 5th ed. Washington, D. C.: American Public Health Association, Inc., 1979.

Review Papers

Atanasiu, P., Avrameas, S., Beale, J., Gardner, P. S., Grandien, M., McIntosh, K., McLean, D. M., Schuurs, A., Sobeslavsky, O., and Voller, A. Progress in the rapid diagnosis of viral infections: a memorandum. *Bull. W.H.O.* 56: 241, 1978.

Herrmann, E. C., Jr. New concepts and developments in applied diagnostic virology. *Prog. Med. Virology* 17: 289, 1974.

Herrmann, E. C., Jr., and Herrmann J. A. Survey of viral diagnostic laboratories in medical centers. *J. Infect. Dis.* 133: 359, 1976.

Hsiung, G. D. Laboratory diagnosis of viral infections: general principles and recent developments. *Mt. Sinai J. Med* 44: 1, 1977.

Hsiung, G. D. Progress in clinical virology 1960–1980—a recollection of twenty years. *Yale J. Biol. Med.* 53: 1, 1980.

Hsiung, G. D., Fong, C. K. Y., and August, M. The use of electron microscopy in diagnosis of viral infection. *Progr. Med. Virol.* 25: 133, 1979.

Nahmias, A. J., and Hall, C. B. Diagnosis of viral diseases—today and tomorrow. *Hospital Practice* 16: 49, 1981.

PART 2: Methods Commonly Used for Virus Isolation and Identification

3. Virus Isolation Methods

Methods for virus isolation vary from laboratory to laboratory. These variations depend not only on the availability of specialized resources and equipment, but also on the animal species and tissue culture systems available. In general, newborn mice, embryonated chicken eggs, and a variety of cell cultures are preferred (figure 3). For arbovirus or coxsackie group A virus infections, newborn mice are the most susceptible hosts. Embryonated eggs are the choice host for influenza A virus; occasionally, certain strains of influenza A virus can be isolated in cell culture. A flowchart outlining the methods for isolating and identifying viruses commonly encountered in a clinical laboratory is provided at the end of this chapter. However, cell cultures remain the most commonly used system in most, if not all, diagnostic virology laboratories.

CELL CULTURE SYSTEMS

Since the discovery that poliovirus multiplies in cultivated animal cells, cell cultures have become the most convenient system for the isolation of many viruses; a variety of primary cell cultures and passaged cell lines are used. While most cell types are available commercially, many can be readily prepared by individual laboratories. Ideally, only freshly prepared cell cultures should be used. Aged cells are frequently less susceptible to virus infection. Table 2 lists the various systems commonly used for the isolation of viruses of the major virus groups. Details of cellular pathology induced by individual viruses are described in separate chapters dealing with the specific virus groups. In general the following procedures apply:

1. Inoculate specimens, 0.1–0.3 ml, into each culture tube. (In selected instances, Leighton tube cultures containing coverslips can be inoculated in a similar manner.)

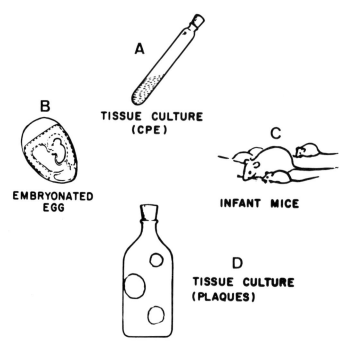

Figure 3. Laboratory techniques for virus isolation.
     A. Tissue culture system for CPE.
     B. Embryonated egg inoculation.
     C. Infant mice inoculation.
     D. Tissue culture system for plaque formation.

2. Check inoculated culture tubes daily for cytopathic effects (CPE). (Certain cell lines, for example Hep-2 cultures, derived from epidermoid carcinoma of the human larynx, require fresh medium changes every 2 days.)
3. When CPE occurs, subculture into a fresh culture of the same cell type to ensure recovery of sufficient virus for identification of the isolate.
4. If CPE is observed in a Leighton tube culture, remove the coverslip with infected cells, wash with phosphate-buffered saline solution (PBS), then fix infected cells on coverslip with Zenker's fixing fluid containing 5% glacial acetic acid for 24 hours or overnight; wash with water and store in 80% ethanol. For immunofluorescence, coverslip cultures should be fixed with dry acetone for 10 minutes and stored at $-20°C$ or $-70°C$. (See p. 60 for reagents and procedures.)

NEWBORN MOUSE INOCULATION

Most group A coxsackieviruses and some togaviruses are isolated best in newborn mice; specimens suspected of harboring these viruses should be inoculated into this animal system. Caution should be taken to avoid errors related to method of inoculation (figure 4).

1. Inoculate newborn mice within 24–48 hours of birth, with 0.01–0.02 ml/mouse intracerebrally, and/or with 0.03–0.05 ml/mouse intraperitoneally, using a 25-gauge ⅜″-long needle and a ½-cc syringe.
2. Check inoculated mice twice daily for signs of illness, paralysis, or death.
3. Harvest mouse brain or skeletal muscle when animals are paralyzed or when other symptoms appear; make 10% tissue suspension and inoculate into appropriate monolayer cell cultures and/or mice for further study.

EMBRYONATED EGG INOCULATION

The chick embryo is a highly sensitive host for primary isolation of several virus types. For certain strains of influenza virus and for mumps virus the amniotic route of inoculation is preferable. On the other hand, chorioallantoic membranes are highly susceptible to pock formation by certain herpes- and poxviruses.

Amniotic or Allantoic Cavity Inoculation

1. Use 7- to 13-day-old embryonated eggs (optimum for mumps, 7–8 days; for influenza, 10–13 days).
2. Candle the eggs and make a puncture through the shell over the air sac.
3. Inoculate 0.1–0.2 ml of the specimen into the amniotic sac and/or allantoic cavity, using a 1¾″-long, 23-gauge needle; use 3 or 4 eggs per specimen. (Note: these procedures should be done under an egg candler; see figure 5A or B.)
4. Seal the hole in the shell with Scotch tape.
5. Incubate eggs at 35°C–37°C with air sac uppermost.
6. Candle inoculated eggs daily. Discard those that die within 24 hours after inoculation.
7. Harvest amniotic fluids (AMF) and allantoic fluids (ALF) separately, 2–4 days after inoculation for influenza and 5–7 days for mumps. The procedure for harvesting egg fluids is as follows:
   a. Chill eggs at 4°C for 2–4 hours.
   b. Open eggshell over the air sac.
   c. Cut out and remove overlying shell membrane and chorioallantoic membrane with scissors.
   d. Aspirate ALF and AMF separately with sterile capillary pipettes.
8. Carry out a spot hemagglutination test by mixing 0.4 ml ALF or AMF and 0.4 ml of a 0.5% suspension of guinea pig red blood cells (RBC). Allow this mixture to stand at room temperature for 30–45 minutes before reading.

Table 2. *In Vitro* and *In Vivo* Systems for Virus Isolation

Virus Family (-viridae)	Virus Type	*In Vitro* Cell Culture System[a]										*In Vivo*	
		Cytopathic Effect in Liquid Medium									Plaque Formation under Agar Medium	Newborn Mice	Embryonated Eggs
		Primary cell culture						Passaged Cell Lines					
		HEK	RhMK or GMK	Patas MK	RK	CE	HDF	Hep-2, HeLa, A549	BSC-1 or Vero	BHK-21			
Picorna-	entero-	++/-	++/-	++/-	-	-	++/-	++/-	++/-	-	+/-	-/++	-
	rhino-	+	+/-	+/-	-	-	++	+/-			+/-	-	-
Toga-	alpha- & flavi-	+/-	+/-	+/-	+/-	++/-			+/-	+/-	++/-	++	+/-
Myxo-	influenza[b]	-	-	← hemadsorption →							+/-	-	++
	parainfluenza[b]	-	-	← hemadsorption →							+/-	-	-
Pseudomyxo-	measles	+	+	← syncytium of intracytoplasmic and intranuclear eosinophilic inclusions →			+/-	+ syn.	syn.		+	-	-
	respiratory syncytial	-	+/-	← syncytium →			-	++ syn.	+/-		+	-	-
Rubi-	rubella	+/-	+/-	-	+/-	-	-	-/+	+/-	+	+	-	-
Reo-	reo-	+	+/-	+/-	+/-	-	+/-	+/-	+/-	+/-	+	-/+	-
Adeno-	adeno-	++	+/-	-	-	-	-	++	-	-	+/-	-	-

← interference with echo-11 → (rubella)

← intracytoplasmic eosinophilic inclusions → (reo-)

← intranuclear basophilic inclusions → (adeno-)

Primary cell culture

Herpes-	herpes-	++	+/-	+/-	+/-	+/-	++	++	+/-	+/-	+/-	+/-
Pox-	pox-(Vaccinia)	+	+	+	+	+	+	+	+/-	+/-	+ (mice & rabbits)	+

— intranuclear eosino- & basophilic inclusions →

— intracytoplasmic Feulgen-positive inclusions →

Primary cell culture
CE   chick embryo fibroblast
GMK   green monkey kidney
HEK   human embryonic kidney
MK   monkey kidney
patas   patas monkey kidney
RhMK   rhesus monkey kidney
RK   rabbit kidney

Diploid cell strain
HDF   human diploid fibroblast
        (including WI-38, IMR-90, MRC-5)

Other cell lines
A549   human lung carcinoma
BHK-21 baby hamster kidney
BSC-1   African green monkey kidney
HeLa   human cervix carcinoma
Hep-2   human larynx carcinoma
Vero   African green monkey kidney

[a]Most of the cell cultures are commercially available.
[b]Hemadsorption positive when RBC added.

Key: + = virus-induced change
        − = no change

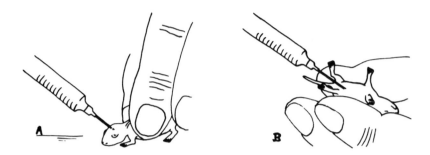

Figure 4. Mouse inoculation.
    A. Intracerebral route.
    B. Intraperitoneal route.

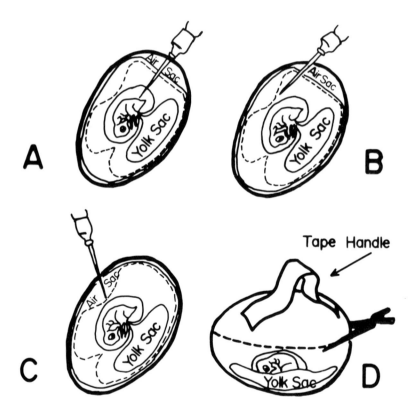

Figure 5. Embryonated egg inoculation and harvesting.
    A. Amniotic cavity inoculation.
    B. Allantoic cavity inoculation.
    C. Chorioallantoic membrane inoculation.
    D. Harvesting chorioallantoic membrane.

Flow Chart for Virus Isolation and Identification[a]

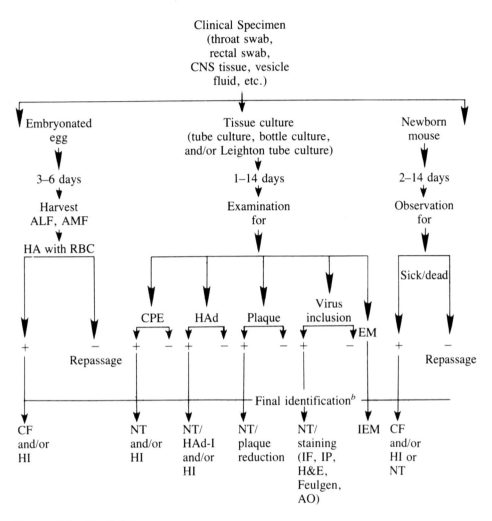

[a]See p. xxii for abbreviations.
[b]Serologic methods of choice for final identification vary according to the virus isolate.

Chorioallantoic Membrane Inoculation and Harvesting

1. Candle eggs containing 9- to 12-day-old developing chicken embryos; mark an area free from large blood vessels on the side where the embryo is located and the area over the air sac.
2. Drill two slits in the eggshell, one on the side and the other over the air sac.

3. Puncture the shell membrane under the slits with a sterile needle; care should be taken not to damage the choriollantoic membrane (CAM).
4. With a rubber bulb, gently apply suction at the hole over the air sac. If this procedure is carried out while the egg is being candled, one can see the CAM drop and a new, artificial air sac form (figure 5C).
5. Place 0.05 ml inoculum on the dropped membrane by inserting the needle through the side slit to a depth of about 5 mm. Withdraw the needle very slowly. Seal the opening with Scotch tape or wax and incubate at 35°C–37°C with the artificial air sac uppermost.
6. Candle the inoculated eggs daily; discard those that die within 24 hours after inoculation.
7. Harvest the CAM as follows:
   a. Place inoculated egg on a holder so that the slit through which the inoculum was delivered faces upward.
   b. Make a tape handle over the area of inoculation (figure 5D).
   c. Cut off top half of the eggshell, including the infected area, and gently remove CAM, which is attached to the shell.
   d. Place infected CAM in a petri dish with a few milliliters of PBS; spread membrane flat against bottom of dish; place dish on a dark surface to facilitate counting of pocks.

4. Virus Assay and Neutralization Test

CYTOPATHIC EFFECT IN CELL CULTURES WITH LIQUID MEDIUM

The rate of cellular change and the pattern of CPE induced by different viruses varies greatly depending upon (a) the type of cell culture system used, (b) the concentration of virus in the specimen, and (c) the properties of each virus strain. Once CPE is obtained, virus infectivity titers can be estimated by the 50% tissue culture infectious dose end point (TCID$_{50}$) originally described by Reed and Muench.

Example

Dilution of virus	No. of cultures showing CPE/no. inoculated	Cumulative no. infected	Cumulative no. not infected	Calculated infectivity Ratio	Percent
10^{-3}	4/4	9	0	9/9	100
10^{-4}	3/4	5	1	5/6	83
10^{-5}	2/4	2	3	2/5	40
10^{-6}	0/4	0	7	0/7	0

In this example the proportionate distance between two dilutions (10^{-4} and 10^{-5}) where the 50% end point lies is equal to:

$$\frac{\text{infectivity above 50\%} - 50\%}{\text{infectivity above 50\%} - \text{infectivity below 50\%}} = \frac{83 - 50}{83 - 40} = 0.7$$

Therefore, a virus suspension of $10^{-4.7}$ per 0.1 ml represents one TCID$_{50}$; that is, at such dilution 50% of the cultures inoculated will become infected. A dilution of $10^{-2.7}$ per 0.1 ml of virus suspension will contain 100 TCID$_{50}$ in a volume of 0.1 ml.

PLAQUE FORMATION IN BOTTLE CULTURES UNDER AGAR OVERLAY MEDIUM

Virus plaques are colorless areas of necrotic cells surrounded by viable cells stained with a vital dye, neutral red. Different animal viruses induce plaques of varying sizes and shapes in much the same manner that different bacteria produce characteristic colonies. Since one infectious virus unit is theoretically capable of initiating one plaque, this technique can be used both for accurate quantitative assay of virus infectivity and for purification of virus strains.

1. Prepare agar overlay medium (for formula, see p. 32).
2. Drain the culture fluids from 7- to 8-day-old culture in 3 oz. prescription bottle or 25-cm^2 culture flask of monkey kidney (or other suitable) cells showing confluent cell sheets.
3. Make serial 10-fold dilutions of virus suspension from 10^{-1} to 10^{-6} and inoculate each into a bottle culture, 0.1–0.5 ml per bottle, and tilt bottle to distribute the inoculum evenly over the entire sheet.
4. Incubate 37°C for 1–2 hours to allow virus adsorption onto monolayer cultures.
5. Add prewarmed agar overlay medium containing neutral red, approximately 8 ml per bottle or 5 ml per 25-cm^2 flask, and lay flat to cover cell sheet.
6. Avoid exposure of inoculated cultures to light after overlay, since photosensitization may injure cultured cells as a result of the presence of neutral red in the overlay medium.
7. Invert culture bottles after agar has solidified and incubate at 37°C in the dark.
8. Check overlaid cultures daily for 2–3 weeks for the appearance of plaques induced by the virus.
9. Pick plaques if present (figure 6) by scraping the areas surrounding the degenerated cells under the agar and within the plaque area with the bent tip of a capillary pipette. Transfer the material from the pipette into a fresh culture tube or a bottle culture to obtain purified virus stock.
10. Plaque size and morphology can be used for characterization of certain virus types, especially within the enterovirus group (see chap. 12).

PLAQUE FORMATION IN PLATE CULTURES UNDER METHYL CELLULOSE OVERLAY MEDIUM

Virus plaques also can be observed in fixed and stained monolayer cultured cells in multiwell plates following incubation under a semisolid overlay medium (figure 7). The plaques can easily be enumerated and the stained plates can be kept permanently.

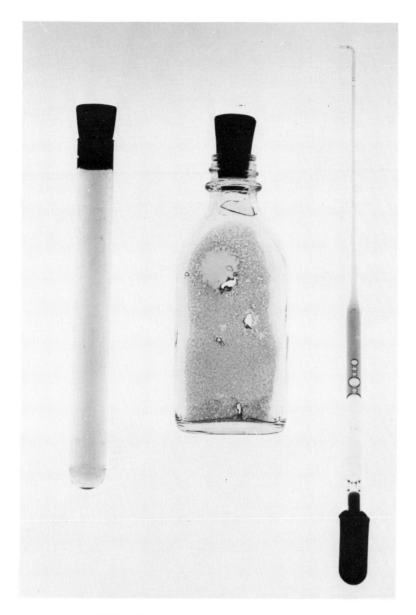

Figure 6. Technique for picking virus plaques in bottle culture. Plaque virus can be subcultured by scraping the degenerated cells under agar and within the plaque area (center of bottle) with the bent tip of a capillary pipette (right) and transferring the material to a fresh culture tube (left) (G. D. Hsiung and J. L. Melnick, *Ann. N.Y. Acad. Sci.* 70: 342, 1958).

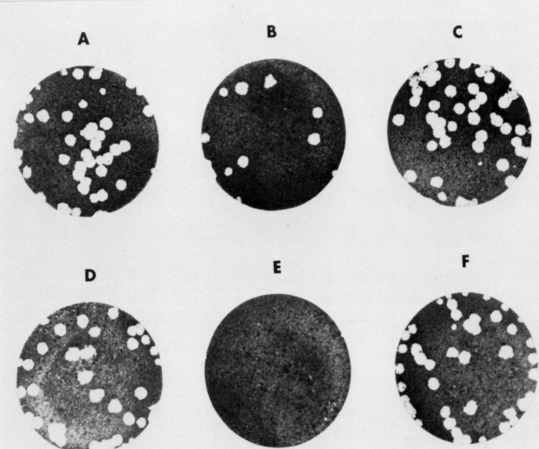

Figure 7. HSV-2 plaque formation in multiwell plastic plate cultures; fixed and stained. Top row: Drug sensitivity assay of HSV-2 plaque formation in guinea pig embryo (GPE) cells, effect of Acyclovir at varying concentrations (in μM) 3 days after incubation (courtesy of A. D. Pronovost). Bottom two rows: Neutralization test of HSV-2 in chicken embryo (CE) cells, 4 days after incubation.

A and D. Virus controls.

B and C. Anti-HSV-1 serum 1:20, 1:40, respectively. Note: plaque reduction at serum 1:20.

E and F. Anti-HSV-2 serum 1:20, 1:40, respectively. Note: complete inhibition of plaques at serum 1:20.

1. Prepare methyl cellulose overlay medium (for formula, see p. 34).
2. Drain the culture fluids from the plates containing confluent cell sheets.
3. Make serial 10-fold dilutions of virus suspension from 10^{-1} to 10^{-6} and inoculate each into a well, 0.1–0.2 ml per well; tilt the plate to distribute the inoculum evenly over the entire cell sheet.
4. Incubate in a 5% CO_2 incubator for 1 hour at 37°C to allow virus adsorption.
5. Add 1% methyl cellulose overlay medium, 1–4 ml per well, depending on size of well.
6. Incubate plates in a 5% CO_2 incubator at 37°C.
7. After 3–10 days (depending upon virus type suspected; for example, 3 days for herpes simplex virus, 10 days for cytomegalovirus) remove the overlay medium by suction.
8. Fix and stain the infected monolayer cultures with a fixative fluid containing 5% formalin and 1.3% crystal violet, 0.5–2 ml per well (for formula, see p. 34). (The entire plate culture can be fixed in 10% formalin prior to staining.)
9. After 20 minutes, wash gently but thoroughly under tap water.
10. Count the number of plaques and calculate virus infectivity titers.

This technique can be used for assaying antiviral agents (figure 7, top row).

NEUTRALIZATION TEST IN CELL CULTURES

There are a variety of serologic tests that are commonly used for virus identification (table 3). The neutralization test (NT) in cell culture is the most sensitive and accurate method for identifying a virus isolate.

Neutralization Test (Inhibition of CPE)

1. Determine virus infectivity titer prior to the test. (For a rapid identification one may select a dilution based on the rapidity with which it induces CPE.)
2. Add equal volumes of a constant virus dilution containing approximately 100 $TCID_{50}$ per 0.1 ml to a known type-specific antiserum at a concentration of 20 units and mix well. (Note: 1 unit equals the highest serum dilution that neutralizes 100 $TCID_{50}$ of virus infectivity.)
3. Allow the virus-serum mixture to remain at room temperature for 1 hour; inoculate 0.2 ml of the virus-serum mixture into each of 2–4 culture tubes.
4. For the virus control, inoculate 0.1 ml of each serial 10-fold dilution into a set of cultures, 2–4 tubes per dilution.
5. Check all tubes for CPE daily for 5–7 days.

Complete inhibition of CPE at a challenge dose of 100 $TCID_{50}$ by a known antiserum type is considered a positive serum neutralization test and indicates the identity of the virus. (It is always advisable to use serum pools, if avail-

Table 3. Serologic Tests Commonly Used for Virus Identification and/or Antibody Determination

Virus Type	Neutralization Tests		Other Serologic Tests	Remarks
	Test System Commonly Used	Method for Testing	Methods	
Enterovirus	MK cell culture	CPE/plaque	HI, CF	HI for certain echovirus types
	newborn mice	sickness/death		mouse for certain coxsackie A virus neutralizations
Rhinovirus	HDF and/or HEK cell culture	CPE		
Togavirus	BHK-21 cell culture and/or Vero cell culture	CPE/plaque	HI, CF, IF	
Rubella virus	Vero cell culture Primary GMK	CPE Interference	HI, CF	
Influenza virus	MK cell culture	HAd	HI, CF	
Parainfluenza virus	MK cell culture	HAd		
Measles virus	Hep-2 cell culture	CPE	CF, HI	
Respiratory syncytial virus	Hep-2 cell culture or A549 cell culture	CPE	CF, IF	
Reovirus	MK cell culture	CPE	HI, CF	

30

Virus			
Rotavirus	None	None	ELISA, IEM, CF	
Rabies virus	BHK-21 cell culture, mouse brain section	IF/plaque	NT	
Adenovirus	Hep-2 cell culture, HEK, A549	CPE/plaque	CF, HI	HI for certain types
Herpes simplex virus	RK cell culture	CPE/plaque	IF, CF	
Varicella-zoster virus	HDF cell culture	CPE	CF	
Cytomegalovirus	HLF cell culture	CPE	CF	slow CPE appearance
Vaccinia virus	MK or CE cell culture	CPE/plaque	HI	selected chick RBC
Hepatitis A virus	None	None	IEM, RIA	IF of liver biopsy
Hepatitis B virus	None	None	RIA, IEM, ELISA, IF, IAH	IF of liver biopsy

Tests

CF	complement-fixation test
ELISA	enzyme-linked immunoabsorbent assay
HAd	hemadsorption
HI	hemagglutination-inhibition test
IAH	immune adherence hemagglutination
IEM	immunoelectron microscopy
IF	immunofluorescent staining
NT	neutralization test
RIA	radioimmunoassay

able, for preliminary identification of an isolate. Final identification can then be confirmed by using type-specific antiserum.)

Neutralization Test (Plaque Reduction)

1. Determine virus infectivity titers by inoculating serial 10-fold dilutions of the virus suspensions into bottle cultures; overlay with nutrient agar and determine plaque counts.
2. Add equal volumes of a constant virus dilution containing approximately 20–50 PFU (plaque-forming units) per 0.1 ml to a known antiserum of 20 units and mix well.
3. Allow the virus-serum mixture(s) and the control virus suspensions in serial 10-fold dilutions to remain at room temperature for 1 hour.
4. Inoculate 0.2 ml of each mixture and 0.1 ml of each control virus dilution into a bottle or flask culture.
5. Incubate bottle or flask cultures at 37°C for 1 hour to allow virus adsorption.
6. Remove bottles from incubator and overlay with prewarmed medium containing agar; avoid exposure to light during and after overlay.
7. Invert bottles after the agar has solidified and incubate at 37°C.
8. Observe the bottle culture daily for the appearance of plaques and make note of their numbers as they appear.
9. An 80% or greater reduction of plaque counts is considered a positive serum neutralization test, and confirms the identity of the virus.

The plaque reduction neutralization test can be carried out in cultures growing in plastic plates by adapting the procedures described above. An example is illustrated in figures 7B and 7E. In selected cases, microtiter plates can be used instead of large-size dishes.

MEDIA AND SOLUTIONS

Agar Overlay Medium for Primary Kidney Cell Culture

A. *Nutrient medium*

	Regular NaHCO$_3$ (ml)	High NaHCO$_3$ (ml)	Low NaHCO$_3$ (ml)
Distilled water, demineralized, sterile	60.0	54.6	63.6
Earle's BSS 10X	18.0	18.0	18.0
Calf serum (heat-inactivated)	3.6	3.6	3.6
NaHCO$_3$ (7.5%)	5.4	10.8	1.8
Neutral red (1:1000)	3.0	3.0	3.0
Penicillin (200,000 units/ml)	0.2	0.2	0.2
Streptomycin (500,000 µ/ml)	0.1	0.1	0.1
Total	90.0	90.0	90.0

Using sterile precautions:

1. Mix each solution according to order listed above.
2. Warm to 37°C in a water bath before use.

B. *Agar*

Agar (Difco-Noble)	2.7 gm
Distilled water, demineralized	90 ml

1. Mix agar with demineralized water and melt in boiling water bath.
2. Autoclave at 15 pounds for 15 minutes.
3. Cool to 43°C before use.

C. *Complete overlay medium*
   When ready for overlay, mix equal volumes of A (nutrient medium) at 37°C and B (3% agar) at 43°C by pouring nutrient medium into the agar; use immediately. After bottles are overlaid, avoid exposure to light.

Agar Overlay Medium for Primary Chicken Embryo Fibroblast Cultures

A. *Nutrient medium*

	(ml)
Distilled water, demineralized, sterile	48.0
Earle's BSS 10X	18.0
Yeast extract (1%)	6.0
Lactalbumin hydrolysate (5%)	6.0
Calf serum (heat-inactivated)	3.6
$NaHCO_3$ (7.5%)	5.4
Neutral red (1:1000)	3.0
Penicillin (200,000 units/ml)	0.2
Streptomycin (500,000 µg/ml)	0.1
Total	90.0

B. *Agar*
   Prepare 3% agar as for regular overlay (see above).

C. *Complete overlay medium*
   When ready for overlay, mix equal volumes of A at 37°C and B at 43°C by pouring nutrient medium into the agar; use immediately. After bottles are overlaid, avoid exposure to light.

Neutral Red (1:1000)

Neutral red (dye content 92%)	1 gm
Distilled water, demineralized	1000 ml

1. Weigh neutral red powder and transfer to a 1-liter volumetric flask.
2. Add demineralized water slowly and mix well until dye dissolves.
3. Make up a final volume of 1000 ml with water.
4. Dispense into smaller convenient volumes.
5. Autoclave at 15 pounds for 15 minutes.
6. Stopper tightly and store at room temperature.

Methyl Cellulose Semisolid Medium

A. *Methyl cellulose solution*

Methyl cellulose powder 4000 centipoise	0.9 gm
Distilled water, demineralized	90 ml

1. Add cold water to methyl cellulose powder, mix well, and autoclave at 15 pounds for 15 minutes; refrigerate. Mixture will be lumpy after autoclaving as methocel liquifies at low temperature and becomes semisolid as the temperature increases.
2. Within the first few hours, constantly shake the flask to dissolve methyl cellulose, which may precipitate a thin layer 12–24 hours after refrigeration. However, it will dissolve completely after 2–3 days at 4°C if it is shaken and mixed often.
3. Be sure all lumps are dissolved before making complete overlay medium.

Note. This medium should be prepared 2–3 days prior to use and kept at 4°C in order to ensure a clear solution.

B. *Nutrient medium*

Distilled water, demineralized	48 ml
Eagle's medium-Earle's with glutamine 10X	18 ml
Calf serum (heat-inactivated)	18 ml
$NaHCO_3$ (7.5%)	6 ml
Antibiotic mixtures	(0.2 ml)
Total	90 ml

Just before use, add solution B to solution A, shaking constantly while pouring.

Fixing and Staining Solutions for Plate Cultures

A. *Crystal violet stock solution (5%)*

Crystal violet powder	25 gm
Absolute ethanol	475 ml

Filter to remove crystals.

B. *Working staining solution (1%)*

Crystal violet (5% stock)	100 ml
NaCl (0.85%)	375 ml
Formalin (formaldehyde 40%)	25 ml

5. Hemagglutination and the Hemagglutination-Inhibition Test

In addition to the neutralization tests described in the previous section, other serologic tests commonly used for virus identification and antibody determination are discussed below and in the following chapters. Table 3 lists the various serologic tests applicable to the representative virus types.

Certain viruses possess the capacity to agglutinate red blood cells (RBC) of specific animal species at defined temperatures (table 4). Specific antibody can be used to prevent this phenomenon.

Preparation of RBC Suspension

1. Obtain blood from guinea pig or other animal or avian species (by cardiac puncture) and mix with either Alsever's solution or heparin to prevent clotting (for Alsever's solution formula, see p. 270).
2. Wash *freshly* obtained RBC three times in PBS and prepare a 10% stock suspension; store at 4°C until used, for no more than one week.
3. Make a 0.5% suspension of the RBC by adding 1 ml of the 10% stock to 19 ml PBS just before use.

TITRATION OF HEMAGGLUTININ

Culture medium from infected cells that exhibit hemadsorption (HAd) may contain virus hemagglutinin that can be assayed by the following procedure:

1. Using either infected tissue culture fluid or infected amniotic-allantoic egg fluid pools, prepare 2-fold serial dilutions (1:10 to 1:640) in PBS in 0.05-ml amounts in disposable microtiter plates. (The amount can be increased if plates with large-size wells are used.)
2. Add 0.05 ml of a 0.5% suspension of guinea pig RBC to each dilution

Table 4. Hemadsorption and Hemagglutination of Viruses with Erythrocytes Obtained from Different Animal Species under Different Conditions

Virus Type	Hemadsorption	Animal Species[a] Erythrocytes Showing Hemagglutination					Optimum Conditions for Erythrocyte Suspension				Serum Treatment
		GP	HO	Chick or Goose	Mon	Rat	Conc.[b] (%)	pH	Diluent	Temp. (C)	
Influenza A, B, C	+	+	+	+[c]	+	+	0.5	7.0	PBS	4°, 22°	RDE and heat adsorption with GP RBC
			←—— elute virus at 37°C ——→								
Parainfluenza 1–5, mumps, NDV	+	+[d]	+	+	+	+	0.5	7.0	PBS	4°, 22°	kaolin treatment adsorption with GP RBC
			←—— elute virus at 37°C ——→								
Measles	+	–	–	–	+	–	0.5	7.0	normal saline	37°	56°C, 30 min. adsorption with monkey RBC
Reovirus	–	+	–	–	–	–	0.75	7.0	normal saline	22°	56°C, 30 min. kaolin treatment
Rubella virus	.–	–	–	+	–	–	0.25	6.2	HSAG[e]	4°, 22°	heparin-MnCl$_2$ treatment adsorption with chick RBC
Adenovirus Group I	–	–	–	–	+	–	0.5	7.2	saline	37°	56°C, 30 min. adsorption with monkey RBC
Group II	–	–	–	–	–	+	0.5	7.0	saline	37°	adsorption with rat RBC

											4°, 22°, 37°	56°C, 30 min. kaolin adsorption
Enterovirus[f]	–	–	+	–	–	–	–	0.5	7.0	PBS		
Togavirus	–	–	–	+		–		0.4	6.0–7.4	borate saline	22°	56°C, 30 min. kaolin adsorption

[a] GP guinea pigs
  HO human type O
  Chick day-old chick
  Mon monkey, preferably African green, reactivity variable from animal to animal; must be preselected
  Rat rats, reactivity variable from animal to animal; must be preselected
[b] RBC suspensions can be standardized spectrophotometrically; variations occur among laboratories.
[c] Chick cells are not agglutinable by new influenza A isolates or certain parainfluenza-type isolates.
[d] Tissue culture fluids from cells infected with parainfluenza virus show low titers of hemagglutinin and are not sufficient for HI test; thus a hemadsorption-inhibition test should be used.
[e] For HSAG formula, see p. 136.
[f] See table 14 for picornavirus types.

Key: + = virus-induced change
     – = no change

of virus suspension and allow the RBC to settle 1–2 hours at 4°C or 22°C. (See table 4 for concentration of RBC, temperature, pH, etc.)

3. Read the virus titer by determining the highest dilution of tissue culture medium (or egg fluid) capable of causing partial or complete hemagglutination (HA). This dilution represents one HA unit (see example below).

Example: Determination of Viral Hemagglutinin Titer

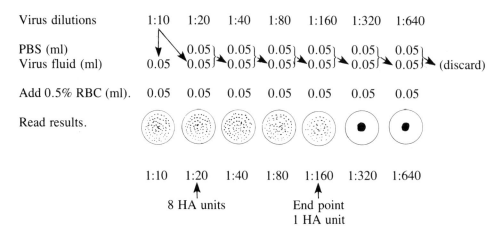

| Virus dilutions | 1:10 | 1:20 | 1:40 | 1:80 | 1:160 | 1:320 | 1:640 |

| 1:10 | 1:20 | 1:40 | 1:80 | 1:160 | 1:320 | 1:640 |

8 HA units   End point
1 HA unit

The HA titer of the virus is 1:160, which represents 1 HA unit. Thus a dilution of 1:20 would contain 8 HA units in 0.05 ml or 4 HA units in 0.025 ml.

Note. The agglutination of RBC in the presence of a myxovirus is due to the adsorption of viral hemagglutinin to glycoprotein receptors present on the surface of erythrocytes. These adsorbed viral particles can be eluted from the RBC at 37°C or after prolonged incubation at room temperature as a result of the presence of viral neuraminidase, which destroys the receptors. However, other viruses, for example the enteroviruses or the adenoviruses, generally do not elute from the RBC after agglutination because of the lack of such enzyme neuraminidase on those virus particles.

HEMAGGLUTINATION-INHIBITION TEST

The HI test is based on the inhibition of viral agglutination by specific serum antibody and can be used for virus indentification and for antibody assay.

Step 1. Determine the viral hemagglutinin units (example described above).
Step 2. Perform the HI test.

1. Make 2-fold serial dilutions in PBS of type-specific antiserum, from 1:10 to 1:640 in 0.025-ml amounts.
2. Add 0.025 ml of the virus dilution containing 4 HA units to each serum dilution.

3. Mix well and allow the virus-serum mixtures to remain for 1 hour at room temperature.
4. Add 0.05 ml of a 0.5% suspension of guinea pig RBC to each mixture; allow to settle for 1–2 hours at 4°C or 22°C.
5. Read the serum titer. The serum titer is the highest dilution of serum-inhibiting hemagglutination by the virus and is expressed as the reciprocal of that serum dilution.
6. To control possible errors in dilution or variations due to different batches of RBC, it is best to back-titrate the 4-HA-unit dilution as in step 3.

Step 3. Back-titrate.
1. Prepare five wells each containing 0.05 ml PBS.
2. To the first add 0.05 ml of test virus dilution containing 8 HA units; mix and transfer 0.05 ml to the second; and continue through the fifth well, discarding the last 0.05 ml.
3. Add 0.05 ml of a 0.5% guinea pig RBC suspension to each well; mix and allow to settle.
4. Only the first three wells should exhibit agglutination, indicating 4 HA units were contained in the 0.025 ml used in the test.
5. Test virus concentration may be adjusted by dilution (with PBS if more than three tubes show agglutination) or by addition of more virus (if less than three tubes show agglutination).

Step 4. Read results.

An example of a type-specific antiserum inhibition reaction is shown below; virus agglutination is inhibited at a serum dilution of up to 1:160.

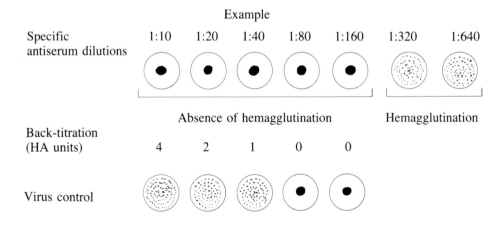

HEMAGGLUTINATION-INHIBITION TEST
FOR ANTIBODY DETERMINATIONS

All serum samples used for the HI test should be heat-inactivated at 56°C for 30 minutes and treated to remove nonspecific inhibitors. Methods for removing nonspecific inhibitors are described below and also under each relevant virus group.

Make serial 2-fold dilutions of acute or convalescent sera in 0.025-ml amounts in PBS using plastic plates; add 0.025 ml of virus suspension containing 4 HA units to each serum dilution. Allow virus-serum mixtures to react at room temperature for 1 hour before the addition of RBC. For diagnostic purposes, a 4-fold or greater HI antibody titer rise is suggestive of recent infection by the test virus or a closely related virus as shown below.

Thus, a 4-fold rise is observed in the convalescent serum (titer = 1:40).

REMOVAL OF NONSPECIFIC INHIBITORS PRESENT IN SERA

In addition to the formulas listed below, other specific treatments are listed within the specific virus group chapters.

Receptor-destroying Enzyme (RDE) Treatment

1. Add 0.4 ml of RDE (100 units per ml) to 0.1 ml serum and incubate at 37°C overnight.

2. Add 0.3 ml of 2.5% sodium citrate to the above mixture and incubate at 56°C for 30 minutes.
3. Add 0.2 ml PBS to the above mixture to yield a final serum dilution of 1:10.

Kaolin Treatment

1. Prepare a 25% suspension of kaolin (acid-washed) in PBS.
2. Mix serum specimen, diluted 1:5 with PBS, with equal volume of the kaolin suspension; shake vigorously and allow to stand at room temperature for 20 minutes, with intermittent shaking.
3. Centrifuge at 2000 rpm for 30 minutes; the supernatant represents the treated serum at a 1:10 dilution.

Trypsin and Periodate Treatment

1. Mix 0.1 ml of 0.8% trypsin solution in PBS with 0.2 ml of undiluted serum and let stand at 56°C for 30 minutes.
2. To this mixture, add 0.6 ml of a 0.01M aqueous potassium periodate solution (255 mg per 100 ml distilled water); allow to stand at room temperature for 15 minutes.
3. Add 0.6 ml of a 1% aqueous glycerol solution and let stand an additional 15 minutes at room temperature.
4. Finally, add 0.5 ml PBS. This final solution gives 2 ml of a 1:10 serum dilution.

REMOVAL OF NATURALLY OCCURRING AGGLUTININS IN SERUM

Certain serum samples contain agglutinins against erythrocytes of foreign species. Therefore, after heat inactivation sera should be diluted 1:5 with PBS and adsorbed with RBC. Add 0.1 ml of the same washed, packed RBC as are to be used for the test to the serum; place the mixture in the refrigerator for 60 minutes and then centrifuge at 4°C at 1500 rpm for 10 minutes; discard the packed cells.

6. Complement-Fixation Test

The complement-fixation (CF) test is a simple and commonly used serologic method for the examination of antibody titers in large numbers of serum specimens as well as for the identification of virus isolates. However, the test is limited in that type-specificity within a virus group usually cannot be determined by this method. There are several procedures, each of which requires some degree of experience. Both the sensitivity and the specificity of the test are affected by the reagents used. A simplified procedure for standardization of the various reagents is described below. More detailed procedures for the diagnostic CF method, designated the Laboratory Branch Complement-Fixation Test or LBCF, are available in a manual prepared by the Laboratory Branch, Center for Disease Control, Atlanta, Georgia.

STANDARDIZATION OF CF REAGENTS

Preparation of Hemolysin Dilutions and Sensitization of Erythrocytes

The incubation of sheep RBC with their homologous antibody is called sensitization. The antibody, hemolysin, is prepared from rabbits immunized with sheep RBC. A stock solution of hemolysin can be prepared at a 1:100 dilution by adding 2 ml of commercially prepared hemolysin in glycerol to 98 ml Veronal buffer (for formula, page 49). This stock can be kept at $-20°C$ in small aliquots for months.

1. From the 1:100 stock hemolysin solution make a 1:1000 dilution. Prepare serial dilutions of the latter using Veronal buffer (VB), as indicated in table 5.
2. Add an equal volume of a 2% washed sheep RBC suspension to each dilution of hemolysin, as shown in table 5 (last two columns).
3. Incubate the mixture at 37°C for 30 minutes to sensitize the RBC.

Table 5. Preparation of Hemolysin Dilutions and Sensitization of Sheep RBC

Dilutions of Hemolysin Desired	Hemolysin Solution (1:1000) (ml)	+	Veronal Buffer (ml)	Discard Excess (ml)	Hemolysin Final Volume (ml)	+	2% Sheep RBC (ml)
1:1000	2.0				2.0		2.0
1:2000	1.0		1.0		2.0		2.0
1:4000	0.5		1.5		2.0		2.0
1:6000	0.4		2.0	0.4	2.0		2.0
1:8000	0.3		2.1	0.4	2.0		2.0
1:10,000	0.2		1.8		2.0		2.0
1:15,000	0.2		2.8	1.0	2.0		2.0
1:20,000	0.2		3.8	2.0	2.0		2.0
1:30,000	0.2		5.8	4.0	2.0		2.0
1:40,000	0.2		7.8	6.0	2.0		2.0

DETERMINATION OF COMPLEMENT UNITS

Commercially prepared complement is usually obtained from "normal" guinea pig sera, which may contain antibody to the test antigen. Complement should therefore be tested for the presence of specific antibody to the virus under test before use. Complement can be obtained commercially in a lyophilized preparation. A 1:10 stock solution is prepared in Veronal buffer and kept in an ice bath during the period of testing.

1. From the 1:10 stock solution make a dilution of 1:50 followed by serial dilutions of complement as shown in table 6; keep in the ice bath.
2. To each 0.2 ml of the various complement dilutions add 0.2-ml amounts of sensitized RBC, either with 2 units of hemolysin if known or with a serial dilultion of hemolysin starting at 1:1000, as shown in table 7.
3. Add 0.2 ml of cold VB to each mixture and incubate for 1 hour at 37°C or overnight in the refrigerator.
4. The highest dilution of complement (1:180 in table 7) at a hemolysin dilution (1:4000, representing 1 unit) giving 100% hemolysis is considered to be a full unit. For identifying viruses, 2 full units of complement should be used in the test. In this case a 1:90 dilution of complement contains 2 units.

CF Test for the Identification of a Virus Isolate in Microtiter Plate

1. Mix 0.025 ml of an unknown antigen (each of the serial dilutions) with 0.025 ml antiserum (each dilution of antiserum) and 0.025 ml complement containing 2 units (see table 8).

Table 6. Preparation of Complement Dilutions

Final Dilutions of Complement Desired	Complement[a] (1:10) (ml)	Veronal Buffer (ml)
1:50	0.5	2.0
1:60	0.4	2.0
1:70	0.4	2.4
1:80	0.3	2.1
1:90	0.3	2.4
1:100	0.3	2.7
1:120	0.2	2.2
1:140	0.2	2.6
1:160	0.2	3.0
1:180	0.2	3.4
1:200	0.2	3.8
1:220	0.2	4.2
1:240	0.2	4.6

[a]Complement obtained commercially is a lyophilized preparation of fresh, normal guinea pig serum and can be reconstituted with 3 ml diluent; a 1:10 stock is prepared in VB and kept *in an ice bath* during the period of use. Stock complement can be stored at $-20°$ for limited periods without appreciable titer loss.

    a. *For antigen control*: 0.025 ml antiserum + 0.025 ml known antigen + 0.025 ml complement.
    b. *For antiserum control*: 0.025 ml VB + 0.025 ml antiserum + 0.025 ml complement.
    c. *For complement control*: 0.025 ml VB + 0.025 ml complement + 0.025 ml unknown antigen; for a back-titration of the complement solution starting with 2 units of complement.
2. Incubate all mixtures in a refrigerator at 4°C overnight.
3. On the following day, remove plates from refrigerator and keep at room temperature for 30 minutes before adding sensitized sheep RBC.
4. In order to sensitize sheep RBC for the indicator system, add 2 units of hemolysin (1:2000) to equal volume of sheep RBC (2%) and mix thoroughly; incubate at 37°C for 30 minutes.
5. Add 0.05 ml of the sensitized sheep RBC to each of the antigen-antiserum mixtures, antigen control, antiserum control, and complement control, and incubate at 37°C for 30 minutes.
6. Record the results as 0 to 4 depending on the degree of fixation of the complement, that is, a 4+ fixation indicates no hemolysis; 0 fixation indicates complete hemolysis.

Table 9 and figure 8 illustrate the results of the CF test for identification of virus isolates. Whenever the titer of an antiserum or a reference serum is known, the block titration shown in table 9 can be omitted and a single serum

Table 7. Determination of Complement Units[a]

Hemolysin Dilutions[b] with Sensitized RBC	Complement Dilutions													Veronal Buffer Only
	50	60	70	80	90	100	120	140	160	180	200	220	240	
1:1000	0	0	0	0	0	0	0	0	0	0	2	2	4	4
1:2000	0	0	0	0	0	0	0	0	0	0	2	2	4	4
1:4000 →	0	0	0	0	0	0	0	0	0	0	2	2	4	4
1:6000	0	0	0	0	0	0	2	2	4	4	4	4	4	4
1:8000	0	0	0	0	0	2	2	4	4	4	4	4	4	4
1:10,000	0	0	0	1	2	2	4	4	4	4	4	4	4	4
1:15,000	0	1	2	2	2	4	4	4	4	4	4	4	4	4
1:20,000	4	4	4	4	4	4	4	4	4	4	4	4	4	4
1:30,000	4	4	4	4	4	4	4	4	4	4	4	4	4	4
1:40,000	4	4	4	4	4	4	4	4	4	4	4	4	4	4

(↑ arrow at 180 column)

[a]Complete hemolysis, 0; 75% hemolysis, 1; 50% hemolysis, 2; 25% hemolysis, 3; no hemolysis, 4. In this test a hemolysin dilution of 1:4000 and a complement dilution of 1:180 completely hemolyzed the sheep cells. Therefore at a 1:4000 hemolysin dilution, 1:180 of complement = 1 unit; 1:90 of complement = 2 units; 1:45 of complement = 4 units. One part of complement is added to 89 parts of VB for 2 units of complement. In this instance, 1 full unit is considered to give 100% hemolysis. Other laboratories may use 50% hemolysis as an end point, making the test more sensitive.
[b]Hemolysin dilutions and 2% sheep RBC are combined in equal volumes for sensitization (see table 5).

Table 8. A Scheme for Complement-Fixation Test in Microtiter Plate

	Unknown Antigen (ml)	Known Antigen (ml)	Antiserum (ml)	VB (ml)	Complement containing 2 units (ml)	Complement unit titration	Sensitized 2% RBC (ml)
Unknown antigen[a] (culture fluid)	0.025	—	0.025	—	0.025		0.05
Known antigen control	—	0.025	0.025	—	0.025		0.05
Antiserum control	—	—	0.025	0.025	0.025		0.05
Complement controls	0.025	—	—	0.025	0.025	(2)	0.05
	0.025	—	—	0.025	0.025	(1)	0.05
	0.025	—	—	0.025	0.025	(½)	0.05
	0.025	—	—	0.025	0.025	(¼)	0.05
Sensitized RBC control	—	—	—	0.075	—		0.05
Buffer (or VB) control	—	—	—	0.050	0.025	(2)	0.05

◄ shake and add ►

◄ overnight at 4°C, following day for 30 minutes at room temp. ►

◄ 1 hour at 37°C ►

[a]Initial antigen or antiserum dilution can be made at 1:2 or 1:4; equal serial dilutions can be made according to the test purpose.

46

Table 9. A Model Complement-Fixation Test[a] for Virus Identification

Antigen Dilutions (Tissue Culture Fluid)	Known Antiserum or Human Reference Serum Dilutions				Antigen Control (No Serum)
	1:16	1:32	1:64	1:128	
1:2	4	4	4	4	0
1:4	4	4	4	4	0
1:8 ◄———	4	4	3	3	0
1:16	2	1	1	1	0
1:32	1	1	0	0	0
1:64	0	0	0	0	0
Serum control (no antigen)	0	0	0	0	
Back-titration of complement	0	0	4	4	
Complement units (0.2 ml)	2	1	½	¼	

[a]Complete hemolysis, 0; 75% hemolysis, 1; 50% hemolysis, 2; 25% hemolysis, 3; no hemolysis, 4. A complete fixation indicates the identity of the virus which has a titer of 1:8 when a known titer of antiserum 1:32 is used. See also figure 8.

dilution (1:32 in table 9) is used for identifying a virus. The highest dilution of the viral antigen that shows 4+ fixation is the titer of the virus isolate.

Interpretation of the Test

The CF test depends on the interaction of antigen, antibody, and complement. If either antigen or antibody is absent, no reaction will occur, and the complement will not be "fixed" and will therefore be free to react with the indicator system, i.e., sheep RBC (antigen), anti-sheep-erythrocyte serum, or hemolysin (antibody). In the latter case, hemolysis of the sheep RBC will occur. Absence (or reduction) of such hemolysis indicates that the complement was fixed by the antigen-antibody combination in the test system. The reactions involved may be presented schematically as follows:

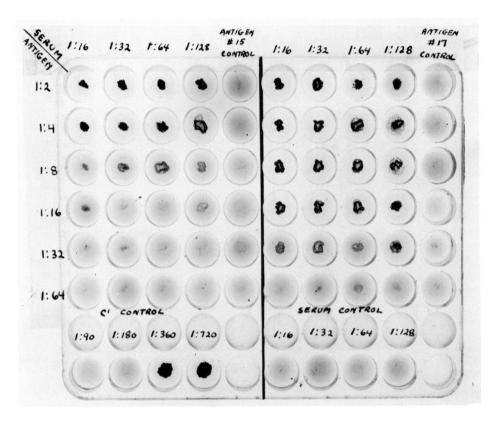

Figure 8. Examples of CF tests in plastic plates with human adenovirus reference serum and two suspected adenovirus isolates. Fixation of complement (C′) = no hemolysis (button of intact RBC); absence of C′ fixation = hemolysis (no button). Titer of antigen 15 (left) is 1:8 and titer of antigen 17 (right) is 1:32; reference serum titer is 1:128.

A Schematic Diagram for a CF Test

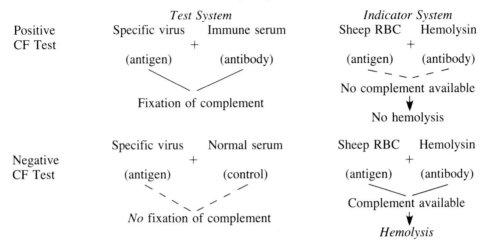

REAGENTS

Veronal Buffer Stock Solution (5X)

Solution A
NaCl	83.80 gm
$NaHCO_3$	2.52 gm
Sodium barbital (sodium 5,5-diethyl barbiturate)	3.00 gm
Distilled water, demineralized	1000 ml

Solution B
Barbital (5,5-diethyl barbituric acid)	4.60 gm
$MgCl_2 \cdot 6H_2O$	1.00 gm
$CaCl_2 \cdot 2H_2O$	0.20 gm
Hot distilled water, demineralized	500 ml

After cooling, add solution A to solution B and bring to 2000 ml with distilled water (5X concentrated). Sterilize by filtration if desired. For a working solution for CF test, to 200 ml of the above mixture add distilled water to 1000 ml (1:5 dilution used as working solution).

7. Enzyme-Linked Immunosorbent Assay (ELISA)

The development of immunoenzymatic methods has greatly advanced diagnostic virology in recent years, both as a means for detecting virus antigens in clinical specimens and for demonstrating viral antibody in serum samples. The use of an enzyme marker provides several distinct advantages, including (1) elimination of the costly and relatively unstable radioisotopes used in radioimmunoassay and (2) the ready standardization of enzyme-antibody conjugates.

In addition to the detection of rotavirus antigen or antibody as described in chapter 17, the ELISA method has been applied to a variety of virus groups, including rubella virus and cytomegalovirus. Schematic diagrams illustrating the direct and indirect ELISA methods for detecting virus antigen and antibody are shown in figures 9 and 10; the procedures are described below.

One disadvantage of the direct ELISA method using a single antiserum approach is that it requires an enzyme-conjugated reagent for each antigen. Therefore, the indirect ELISA method using an unconjugated antiserum, which is subsequently quantitated by the use of an enzyme-labeled anti-immunoglobulin, is more convenient and provides greater flexibility. Furthermore, a number of laboratories have demonstrated that the indirect ELISA provides increased sensitivity over the direct method.

ELISA METHOD FOR ANTIGEN DETECTION

Indirect Method, Using Rotavirus as an Example

1. Precoat round-bottomed polyvinyl microtiter plates. Add 0.1 ml of goat antihuman rotavirus antiserum diluted to 1:20,000 in carbonate buffer to each well (capture antibody). Store at 4°C until use (for at least 24 hours). Wash 3 times in PBS-Tween 20 immediately before use.
2. Add .05 ml of stool extract (2%–10%) and 0.05 ml of PBS-Tween 20

DIRECT METHOD

STEP 1   STEP 2   STEP 3   STEP 4

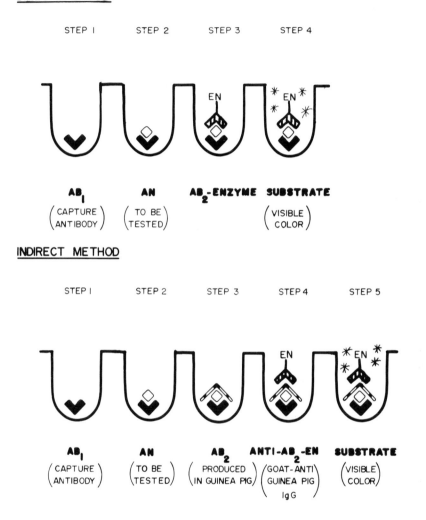

Figure 9. Scheme for ELISA; direct method and indirect method for antigen detection.

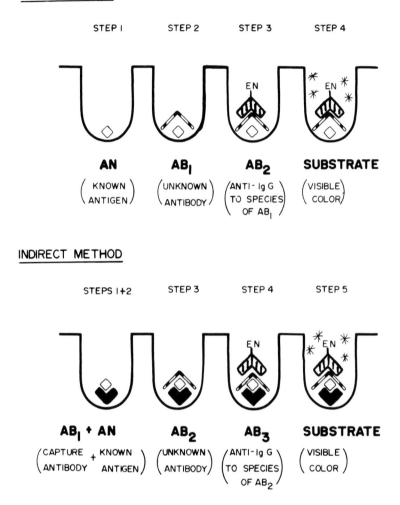

Figure 10. Scheme for ELISA; direct method and indirect method for antibody detection.

52

containing 1% fetal bovine serum and 0.5% goat serum. Incubate at 4°C overnight or at 37°C two hours. Wash 3 times with PBS-Tween 20.

3. Add 0.1 ml of guinea pig antirotavirus serum diluted to 1:500 in PBS-Tween 20 containing 1% fetal bovine serum and 0.5% normal goat serum. Incubate for 1 hour at 37°C. A higher dilution of guinea pig antiserum may be tried (depending on the concentration of virus antigen in the specimen). Wash 3 times with PBS-Tween 20.

4. Add 0.1 ml of alkaline phosphatase-labeled goat anti–guinea pig serum diluted to 1:400 in PBS-Tween 20 containing 1% fetal bovine serum and 0.5% normal goat serum. Incubate at 37°C for 1 hour. Wash 3 times with PBS-Tween 20.

5. Add 0.1 ml of substrate solution (1 tablet containing 5 mg of p-nitrophenyl phosphate disodium to each 5 ml of 10% diethanolamine buffer).

6. Incubate at room temperature until yellow color appears or check results with a spectrophotometer. (Compare yellow color with positive standard or dilution of positive controls.) Add 0.05 ml of 3N NaOH to each well to stop the reaction.

Note. In order to obtain uniform results, only the 60 inner wells of a 96-well microtiter plate are used for test antigens. Fill outer wells with PBS-Tween 20 at each step to ensure even heat distribution.

ELISA METHOD FOR ANTIBODY DETECTION

Indirect Method, Using Rotavirus as an Example

1. Precoat microplate with goat antirotavirus serum diluted to 1:10,000 in carbonate buffer, pH 9.6, 0.2 ml per well. Incubate at least overnight at 4°C (capture antibody).

2. Wash plate with PBS-Tween 20; add rotavirus antigen diluted in PBS-Tween 20. Incubate for 2 hours at 37°C or overnight at 4°C. Store plates at 4°C with the antigen in them. (*Note*: Antigen should be a 2%–10% bacteria-free stool filtrate or suspension stored with 0.2% sodium azide. The optimal dilution should be predetermined by checkerboard titration.)

3. Wash plate before use and add test serum (human serum) in PBS-Tween 20 containing 1% fetal bovine serum and 0.5% normal goat serum, free of rotavirus antibody; the human serum mixture can be diluted to 1:100, 1:400, 1:1600 in the precoated plate. Incubate for 2 hours at 37°C or overnight at 4°C.

4. Wash plate. Add 0.1 ml alkaline phosphatase-labeled goat antihuman IgG diluted in PBS-Tween 20 with 1% fetal bovine serum and 0.5% normal goat serum. Incubate 1–2 hours (depending on conjugate) at 37°C.

5. Wash, add 0.1 ml of prepared substrate solution (p-nitrophenyl phosphate disodium in diethanolamine buffer). Incubate at room temperature for 30

minutes. Add 0.05 ml of 3N NaOH to each well to stop the reaction. Compare yellow color with positive controls. The end point is recorded as the highest serum dilution having a visual color or the highest serum dilution indicating an absorbence reading of 0.75 or greater.

REAGENTS

Carbonate-Bicarbonate Buffer (pH 9.6)

Na_2CO_3	1.59 gm
$NaHCO_3$	2.93 gm
Distilled water, demineralized	1000 ml

Store at 4°C for not more than two weeks.

PBS-Tween 20 (pH 9.6)

NaCl	8.0 gm
KH_2PO_4	0.2 gm
Na_2HPO_4	1.15 gm
KCl	0.2 gm
Distilled water, demineralized	1000 ml
Tween 20	0.5 ml

Store at 4°C.

Substrate Solution

P-nitrophenyl phosphate disodium (1 tablet)	5 mg
Diethanolamine buffer (10%)	5 ml

8. Light Microscopy

Microscopic examination of fixed and stained infected cells is a technique that should not be overlooked in the diagnostic laboratory; it is good practice to include coverslip preparations of cell cultures in selected cases. When cultured cells are stained and mounted, these preparations are a distinct aid in recognizing and identifying viruses and can be filed for reference and become part of the permanent record.

IMMUNOPEROXIDASE STAINING

The immunoperoxidase (IP) staining technique can be used to identify the presence of viral antigen (using a known antiserum) or demonstrate the presence of viral antibody (using a known virus-infected cell culture). The method is analogous to immunofluorescence (IF) and both direct and indirect techniques can be applied. In the IP test, permanent stained preparations can be obtained and examined under a light microscope.

Indirect Staining Method

1. Wash infected cells with PBS with 2 or 3 changes (infected cultures must be treated with caution).
2. Fix cells or tissue sections with acetone for 10 minutes.
3. Treat fixed infected cells or tissue sections with H_2O_2-methanol solution (formula below) for 45 minutes to remove endogenous peroxidase. (If tissue sections are in paraffins, use xylene for 5 minutes, then 100% ethanol, two changes each, before treatment.)
4. Hydrate in 100% alcohol, then 95%, 70%, and 50%, and finally in water, two changes each; wash in PBS (for PBS formula, see p. 268, but omit calcium and magnesium salts).

55

5. *If paraffin tissue sections are used*, treat with 0.25% trypsin in PBS containing 0.02% $CaCl_2$ for 30 minutes.
6. Overlay with 1:10 or 1:20 normal rabbit serum (or other serum of the same host species for the second antibody) for 30 minutes; remove excess serum. To dilute normal serum, use PBS-BSA (bovine serum albumin) diluent (see formula below).
7. Add human antibody (or antibody of other species to be tested) diluted with PBS-BSA at 37°C for 1–2 hours or overnight at 4°C; remove excess serum (human serum in this case) and wash in PBS 3 changes.
8. Add rabbit antihuman IgG-peroxidase conjugate (1:50 diluted with PBS-BSA) for 30 minutes; wash with PBS 3 changes.
9. Add freshly prepared 0.05% DAB solution (formula below) for 5–10 minutes or until brown color appears.
10. Remove substrate; wash with PBS and water.
11. Counter stain with hematoxylin if needed.
12. Dehydrate in ethanol 50%, 70%, 95%, and 100% and clarify in xylene.
13. Mount on microscopic slides with mounting medium (Permount or Harleco synthetic resin).
14. Examine stained preparation with a light microscope (see figure 70).

Reagents for Immunoperoxidase Staining

H_2O_2-Methanol Solution

H_2O_2 (30%)	3	ml
Methanol	97	ml

PBS-BSA Diluent

PBS	100	ml
Bovine serum albumin	4	gm

DAB Solution (to be prepared just before use)

DAB (3,3'-diaminobenzidine tetrahydrochloride)	5	mg
Distilled water, demineralized	10.00	ml
H_2O_2 (30%)	0.05	ml

HEMATOXYLIN-EOSIN STAINING

The structure of the cell is often altered to a greater extent by Zenker's fixing solution than by formalin, since the chromatin often appears as a coarse reticulum and the cytoplasm is somewhat foamy. However, Zenker's fixing solution is particularly useful for the demonstration of virus-induced intranuclear inclusions, and thus preserves sharp structural details of virus-infected cells.

Procedure

1. Wash infected cultures in PBS with 3 changes (infected cultures must be treated with caution).
2. Fix cells on coverslips in Zenker's fixing solution for 24 hours or overnight at room temperature.
3. Wash in cold running water until the water is clear.
4. Dehydrate in 80% ethanol, or store in 80% ethanol if samples are not to be stained immediately.
5. Dip in alcohol iodine (0.5% iodine in 95% ethanol) for 1 minute to remove mercury precipitate; rinse in water.
6. Dip in 0.5% aqueous sodium thiosulfate for 1 minute to remove excess iodine, if any; rinse in water.
7. Stain in hematoxylin for 1–2 minutes; rinse in water.
8. Differentiate in 1% ammonium hydroxide solution for 3–5 seconds or until a blue color appears; rinse in water.
9. Counterstain with 0.5% eosin in 95% ethanol for 1–2 minutes.
10. Dehydrate rapidly in two changes of 100% ethanol.
11. Clear in 2 changes of xylene, 1 minute each.
12. Mount on microscope slides with cell side down using mounting medium (Permount or Harleco synthetic resin).
13. Clean upper surface of coverslip, after mounting medium has set for 24 hours, in order to remove cells or debris that may have adhered to the upper surface of the coverslips.
14. Examine stained preparations with a light microscope (see color figures 1, 2, 3, 5, 7, and 8).

Reagents for Hematoxylin-Eosin Staining

Zenker's Fixing Solution

Potassium dichromate	2.5 gm
Mercuric bichloride	5.0 gm
Distilled water, demineralized	100.0 ml

This solution should be dissolved with the aid of heat. This stock solution keeps very well; just before using, add glacial acetic acid to 5%.

Harris Hematoxylin

Distilled water	200 ml
Hematoxylin	1 gm
Absolute ethanol	10 ml
Ammonium or potassium aluminum sulfate	20 gm
Mercuric oxide (red)	0.5 gm

Dissolve the hematoxylin in the alcohol and the aluminum sulfate in water with the aid of heat. Combine the hematoxylin and the alum solutions and bring to a boil as rapidly as possible. Then add the mercuric oxide. The solution takes on a dark or purple color. Transfer the flask to a cold-water bath. This solution does not need the addition of ripening agents and can be used as soon as it is cold, although better staining results are obtained if it is made a few days in advance. Filter before using or storing. Keep in a tightly stoppered bottle. This and other hematoxylin staining solutions may be purchased commercially.

Eosin

Eosin Y, both water- and alcohol-soluble, gives good results. A 0.5% to 1% solution of eosin, either in water or 95% ethanol, should be used. The solution must be filtered before use.

FEULGEN REACTION

Carnoy's fluid is recommended for cell fixation prior to the use of Feulgen reagent.

1. Wash infected cultures in PBS (3 changes).
2. Fix cells on coverslips in Carnoy's solution for 20 minutes.
3. Transfer to 95% ethanol for 2 minutes.
4. Transfer to 70% ethanol for 2 minutes.
5. Wash in water for 2 minutes.
6. Transfer to HCl (1N) and leave for 2 minutes.
7. Then transfer to HCl (1N) prewarmed to 60°C and keep at 60°C for 10–20 minutes.
8. Transfer to room temperature HCl (1N) for 2 minutes.
9. Wash quickly in water.
10. React with Schiff's reagent for 30 minutes.
11. Wash in running water for 5–15 minutes or until free from unbound reagent.
12. Counterstain with light green (0.5%) if desired, and wash in water.
13. Rapidly dehydrate in 70% ethanol, 2 minutes.
14. Rapidly dehydrate in 95% ethanol (2 changes).
15. Rapidly dehydrate in 100% ethanol (2 changes).
16. Transfer to xylene.
17. Mount on slides and examine under light microscope.

A Feulgen-positive reaction, the presence of a red color after reacting with Schiff's reagent, indicates the presence of DNA. See color figure 6.

Carnoy's Fixing Fluid

Absolute ethanol	6 ml
Chloroform	3 ml
Glacial acetic acid	1 ml

Prepare fresh each time. This is one of the best fixatives for Feulgen stain reaction.

Schiff's Reagent

1. Add 200 ml boiling distilled water to 1 gm basic fuchsin.
2. Cool to 50°C and filter.
3. Add 20 ml 1N HCl and cool to room temperature.
4. Add 2 gm potassium metabisulfate ($K_2S_2O_5$). Allow to stand overnight.
5. If not straw-colored on the following day, add a pinch (about 0.5 gm) of charcoal; shake and filter after 1 minute.
6. Store in refrigerator. The reagent may be used repeatedly until it turns pink.

9. Dark-Field Microscopy

IMMUNOFLUORESCENT STAINING

The immunofluorescent (IF) staining technique has been used for the rapid diagnosis of viral diseases and for the investigation of a variety of virus-cell systems. At present the prompt diagnosis of rabies virus infection is commonly made by the IF test. Techniques of fixation and staining may vary according to the specific virus cell–antibody system under study. Modifications of standard techniques may be necessary. For satisfactory results, high titers of specific antiserum and/or high concentrations of antigen are essential.

Direct Staining Method

1. Wash coverslips containing infected or uninfected cells with PBS, 2 or 3 changes (infected cultures must be treated with caution); dry at room temperature.
2. Fix with dry acetone for 10 minutes; dry at room temperature (at this step the fixed cells on coverslips can be stored at $-20°C$ in stoppered tubes for later use).
3. Overlay infected cells on coverslips with fluorescein-labeled antiserum. Let stand 30 minutes at 37°C or room temperature in petri dish containing moist gauze.
4. Wash in PBS to remove excess labeled antiserum (3 changes); dry coverslips at room temperature.
5. Mount with buffered glycerin (1 ml PBS + 9 ml glycerin that has been prepared within a 3-week period).
6. Cover with a 22 mm $\times$ 50 mm (00 thickness) coverslip and seal with colorless nail polish to prevent evaporation.
7. Examine the preparations under a microscope with a dark-field condenser and UV light source.

Indirect Staining Method

Steps 1 and 2 are the same as for the direct method.

3. Overlay infected cells on coverslips with unlabeled antiserum (e.g., that produced in rabbits) and let stand for 30 minutes in a petri dish containing a piece of moist gauze (as controls, normal rabbit serum can be used instead of antiserum).
4. Wash off excess antiserum with PBS (3 changes); dry coverslips at room temperature.
5. Add fluorescein-labeled antiglobulin (in this instance, antirabbit globulin produced in goats) and let stand to react with the rabbit antiserum that was added in step 3 for 30 minutes in a covered petri dish containing moist gauze.
6. Wash off excess labeled antiglobulin with PBS (3 changes); dry coverslips at room temperature.
7. Mount with buffered glycerin and cover with 22 mm × 50 mm (00 thickness) coverslips; examine under a dark-field microscope with UV light source.

Interpretation of Results

The specificity of fluorescent staining of virus-infected cells may be difficult to determine without proper controls. The absence of fluorescent staining in uninfected cells, or in infected cells with normal rabbit serum, is a good indication that the results are specific.

Figure 11 illustrates schematically the direct and indirect fluorescent labeling reaction. Direct staining of virus aggregates in infected cells using labeled antibody generally does not present serious difficulties in interpretation, provided the labeled antibody is of high titer, does not cause nonspecific staining, and shows no or very limited amounts of cross-staining reaction with heterologous antigens. An example of a direct IF–stained preparation of RhMK cells infected with reovirus type 1 is shown in figure 58. An example of the indirect staining method is shown in figure 59.

The indirect method can be employed to simplify the identification of antigens. In this system, an antiglobulin is labeled and used as an indicator for the antigen-unlabeled antibody complex. For example, if an antibody used in the primary reaction is prepared in rabbits, a labeled antirabbit globulin prepared in goats could be used to detect rabbit globulin present in the primary reaction. That is, the unlabeled antibody plays a dual role, acting as an antibody in the primary reaction and as an antigen in the secondary reaction.

DIRECT METHOD

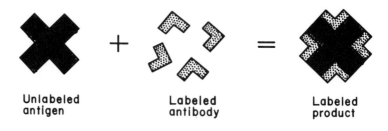

| Unlabeled antigen | Labeled antibody | Labeled product |

INDIRECT METHOD

STEP 1:

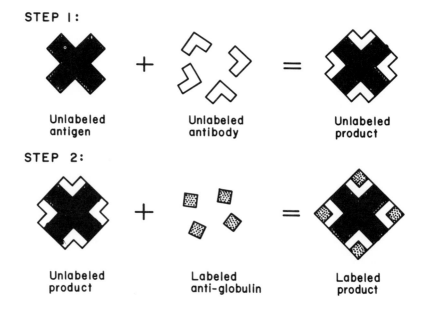

| Unlabeled antigen | Unlabeled antibody | Unlabeled product |

STEP 2:

| Unlabeled product | Labeled anti-globulin | Labeled product |

Figure 11. Scheme for immunofluorescent staining; direct and indirect methods for antigen or antibody detection.

Table 10. Acridine Orange Staining Properties of Different Virus-Infected Cells

Virus Nucleic Acid	Virus Type	Viral Inclusion	Acridine Orange Staining	Nuclease Susceptibility	
				DNAase	RNAase
Single-stranded RNA	measles virus	nucleus & cytoplasm	flame red	−	+
Double-stranded RNA	reovirus	cytoplasm	yellow-green	−	+
Single-stranded DNA	parvovirus	nucleus	flame red	+	−
Double-stranded DNA	adenovirus	nucleus	yellow-green	+	−
	herpesvirus	nucleus	yellow-green	+	−
	poxvirus	cytoplasm	yellow-green	+	−

ACRIDINE ORANGE STAINING

The acridine orange staining technique can be used for differentiation of DNA and RNA components of a cell. This method can be adapted for the differentiation of a double-stranded DNA or RNA virus from the single-stranded DNA or RNA virus in an infected cell (table 10). The double-stranded DNA or RNA generally shows up as a yellowish green fluorescence; the single-stranded RNA or DNA is orange-red. Better differentiation is obtained if every solution including buffers in the following steps contains 0.002M $MgSO_4$.

1. Wash infected cultures with PBS, 2 or 3 times (care should be taken in discarding PBS that contains infectious virus).
2. Fix infected cells on coverslip in freshly prepared Carnoy's fluid for 2–5 minutes (for formula, see p. 59).
3. Hydrate rapidly by immersing coverslips successively in 95%, 80%, 70%, and 50% ethanol, approximately 1 minute each.
4. Rinse in 0.002M $MgSO_4$ solution, approximately 1 minute.
5. Place in 1% acetic acid for 1 minute.
6. Rinse in 0.002M $MgSO_4$ solution for 1 minute.
7. Rinse in phosphate buffer containing 0.067M Na_2HPO_4 and KH_2PO_4 at pH 6.0 for 2 minutes.
8. Stain in 0.01% acridine orange solution prepared in the same phosphate buffer, pH 6.0, for 3 minutes.
9. Rinse in the same phosphate buffer at pH 6.0 for 2–5 minutes.
10. Differentiate in 0.1M $CaCl_2$ containing 0.002M $MgSO_4$ for 2 minutes.
11. Rinse in phosphate buffer, pH 6.0.
12. Mount in the same buffer, cover the stained coverslip with 00 thickness coverslip and seal with nail polish.
13. Examine the preparation in a dark-field microscope with UV light source.

An example of an acridine-orange-stained preparation is shown in color figure 4. Double-stranded reovirus RNA stains green in the cytoplasm, whereas single-stranded cellular RNA stains red in the cytoplasm. Double-stranded cellular DNA stains green in the nucleus (see table 10).

REAGENTS

Potassium Sodium Phosphate Buffer (0.067M), pH 6.0

1. Dissolve 9.465 gm Na_2HPO_4 in 1000 ml distilled water.
2. Dissolve 9.072 gm KH_2PO_4 in 1000 ml distilled water.
3. Mix 40 ml Na_2HPO_4 and 230 ml KH_2PO_4 solution.

Acridine Orange (AO) Solution

1. Stock solution (0.1%): dissolve 0.1 gm of AO powder in 100 ml distilled water (E. Gurr's Microme AO powder obtained from K & K Laboratories, Inc., Plainview, N. Y., gives excellent results).
2. Staining solution (0.01%): dilute 1 ml AO stock solution to 9 ml of 0.067M phosphate buffer, pH 6.0.

Calcium Chloride Solution (0.1M)

Dissolve 11.099 gm $CaCl_2$ in 1000 ml distilled water.

$MgSO_4$ Stock Solution (0.2M)

Dissolve 4.93 gm $MgSO_4 \cdot 7H_2O$ in 100 ml distilled water.

To obtain a 0.002M $MgSO_4$ solution, add 0.1 ml of stock solution to 9.9 ml distilled water.

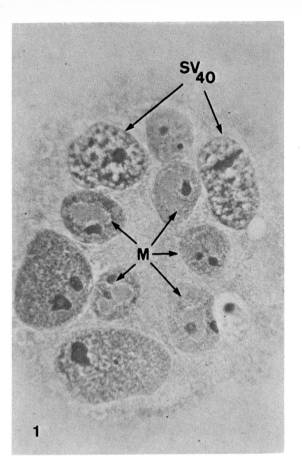

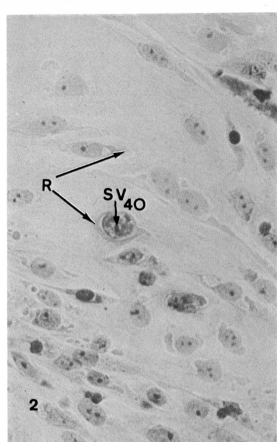

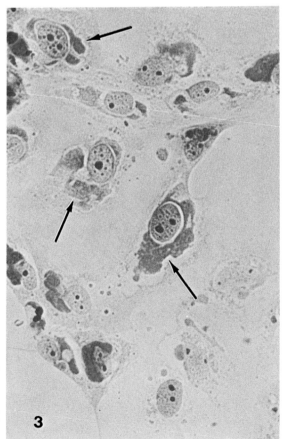

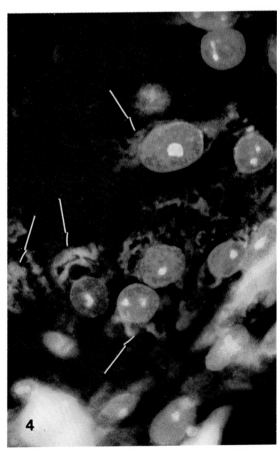

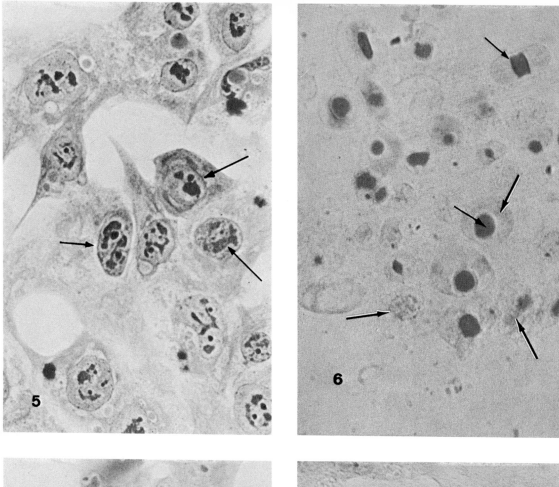

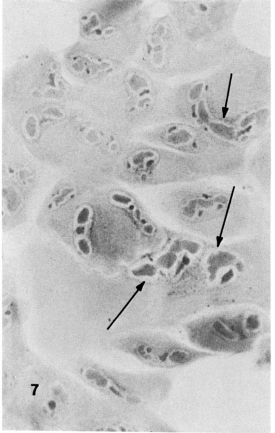

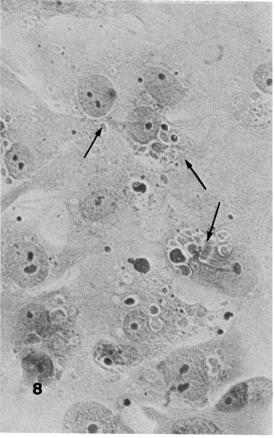

COLOR FIGURES

1. Mixed infection with measles and SV_{40} in a lot of GMK cell culture. Note the eosinophilic intranuclear inclusions induced by measles (M) virus and the basophilic intranuclear inclusions induced by SV_{40} within a multinucleated syncytial cell (H&E, 970X).
2. Mixed infection with reovirus type 1 and SV_{40} in a lot of RhMK cell culture, showing eosinophilic cytoplasmic inclusions induced by reovirus (R) and basophilic nuclear inclusions induced by SV_{40} (H&E, 400X).
3. Eosinophilic cytoplasmic inclusions induced by reovirus type 3 in RhMK cells (H&E, 400X).
4. Greenish cytoplasmic inclusions induced by reovirus type 1 in RhMK cells following acridine orange staining indicating double-stranded RNA (AO, 400X).
5. Basophilic intranuclear inclusions induced by adenovirus type 2 in HEK cells (H&E, 400X).
6. Feulgen-positive intranuclear inclusions induced by an adenovirus in RhMK cells (400X).
7. Eosinophilic intranuclear inclusions induced by human cytomegalovirus in HDF cells (H&E, 400X).
8. Eosinophilic cytoplasmic inclusions induced by vaccinia virus in RhMK cells (H&E, 400X).

10. Electron Microscopy

The recognition of virus particles in clinical specimens by means of electron microscopy (EM) has been made for over 30 years. However, the preparation of the specimens has been considered a tedious and time-consuming task. In recent years, improved technology has simplified many of the procedures and reduced the time needed for processing specimens.

Essentially there are two basic techniques available for routine use: negative staining of virus particles and thin-sectioning of virus-infected cells. Negative staining of clinical material provides the simplest and most rapid method for the detection and recognition of virus particles. Thin-sectioning, although less rapid, provides a more reliable diagnosis, since the examination of virus-infected cells reveals the site of virus replication. In the following sections the two basic techniques for preparing samples for electron microscopy are described.

NEGATIVE STAINING METHOD

The negative staining technique for visualization of virus particles was introduced in 1959 by Horne and Wildy, who described the use of heavy metal salts for enhancing the contrasts in virus-particle images. The procedures are simple and need no special equipment.

1. Mix virus in aqueous suspension with an equal volume of a heavy metal salt solution (2%–4%), such as potassium phosphotungstate acid (PTA) or 0.5% uranyl acetate.
2. Place a drop of the mixture on a Formvar or collodion-coated electron-microscope grid.
3. Remove the excess fluid by blotting with filter paper and air-dry the specimen.
4. Examine the grid containing the mixture under an electron microscope.

The virus particles are surrounded by heavy metal atoms and are revealed against a dark background, the so-called "negative stain," since the electron beam can pass through the low electron density of the virus but not through the metallic background.

However, most clinical specimens contain small numbers of virus particles. Two procedures have been developed for concentration of virus particles and are commonly used in diagnostic laboratories. These are pseudoreplica and agar-diffusion-filtration methods. In addition, immunoelectron microscopy, which was first developed in conjunction with detection of rotavirus particles in stool specimens, has emerged as an extremely useful means for both concentrating virus particles and providing a presumptive diagnosis.

Pseudoreplica Method

This technique was first described by Sharp and has been widely used among viral morphologists and clinical virologists for rapid diagnosis of viral diseases. The procedures are illustrated in figure 12.

1. Place a drop of virus suspension onto a block of 2% agar or agarose on a microscope slide and, under an ultraviolet light, allow the aqueous solution to be diffused and absorbed into the agar for approximately 15 minutes or until dry.
2. Add a drop of 0.5% Formvar solution on the top of the dried virus specimen; drain off the excess Formvar solultion. (This step allows a Formvar membrane to coat the virus specimen on the agar surface.)
3. Trim the excess Formvar membrane with a blade.
4. Immerse the virus-Formvar agar block, at an angle, into a staining jar containing 2% PTA solution (the virus-Formvar membrane will float on the surface of the PTA solution, allowing the staining to take place).
5. Place an electron-microscope grid (300 or 400 mesh) on the virus-Formvar membrane.
6. Pick up grid by a metal peg or with paraffin film. The grid is ready for electron-microscopic examination.

Agar-Diffusion-Filtration Method

This method was first described by Anderson and Doane. It is similar to the pseudoreplica method but simpler to use. The procedures are illustrated in figure 13.

1. Place a 1%–2% agar block on a microscope slide; add a small drop of virus suspension on the surface of the agar block.
2. Place 1 or 2 EM grids (carbon-Formvar coated, 300 mesh) over the drop of virus suspension, upside down, and allow the aqueous solution and salts to diffuse into the agar until the suspension is dry, thus leaving

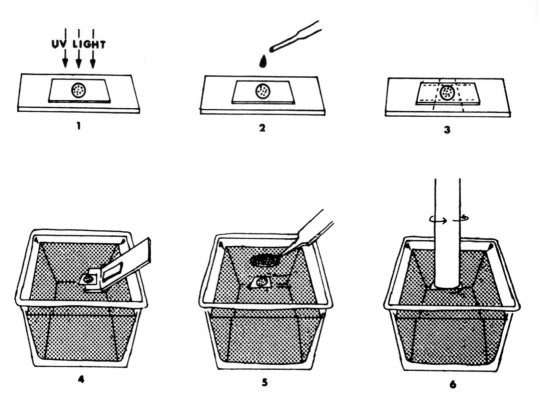

Figure 12. Scheme for pseudoreplica method for preparing specimen for EM examination.

STEP 1

STEP 2

STEP 3

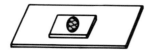

Figure 13. Scheme for agar-diffusion-filtration method for preparing specimen for EM examination.

the concentrated virus particles on the agar surface where they have adhered to the coated grids.

3. Pick up the grids with the virus specimen and stain with 2% PTA solution for 1–2 minutes; remove excess PTA solution by blotting with a filter paper. Examine the grid under an electron microscope.

IMMUNOELECTRON MICROSCOPY

Immunoelectron microscopy (IEM) has been used for rapid serodiagnosis of virus infection or for enhancing concentration in order to facilitate recognition of the relatively small number of virus particles in the specimen. IEM has been widely used for recognizing rotaviruses or Norwalk agent in stool samples of patients with gastroenteritis, and to detect hepatitis B virus surface antigen in patient serum. The procedures are as follows:

1. Mix virus suspension with homologous antiserum at 1:10–1:100 dilutions for 30–60 minutes at 37°C or room temperature to permit formation of virus-antibody aggregates.
2. Centrifuge the virus-antiserum mixtures at 15,000 rpm for 30 minutes.
3. Resuspend the pellet in a small amount of distilled water; mix a drop of this concentrated suspension with a drop of 4% PTA.
4. Apply the stained, concentrated virus-antibody complex to a Formvar-coated EM grid for examination.

Alternatively, after step 1, the virus-antiserum mixture can be placed directly on an agar block and processed by pseudoreplica method or agar-diffusion-filtration method as described above, without ultracentrifugation. IEM is most useful for recognition and identification of those viruses that cannot be easily cultivated in cell cultures, such as rotaviruses (figure 60).

THIN-SECTIONING METHOD

The thin-sectioning method is used to prepare fixed and embedded tissues or cells for electron microscopy; it is more time-consuming and requires personnel with special skills. However, examining the well-preserved virus-infected cells offers the advantage of direct observation of virus-cell interaction, which in turn reveals the site of virus replication and maturation in the host cells, thus aiding in identification of unknown viruses. The conventional procedure consists of primary fixation (with glutaraldehyde or paraformaldehyde), post-fixation (osmium tetroxide), *en bloc* staining with uranyl acetate (optional), dehydration (ethanol or acetone), infiltration (propylene oxide or other solvents), embedding (epoxy resin or other embedding media), thin-sectioning, and staining. The choice of reagents for fixing and embedding varies from laboratory to laboratory and usually depends on experience. For detailed information concerning the use of various buffer solutions, fixatives, and embedding media, the reader is re-

RNA VIRUSES

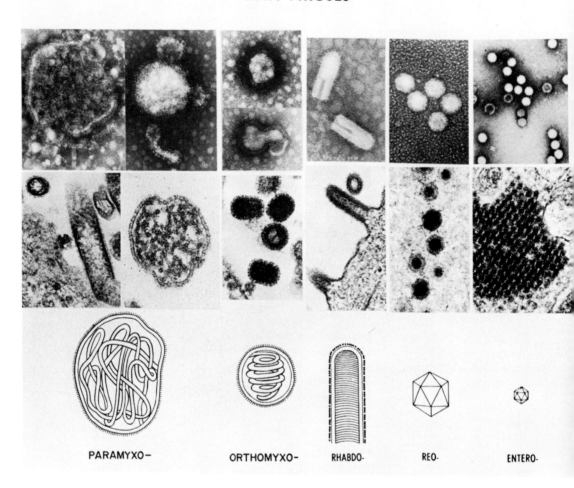

Figure 14. Relative size and shape of RNA viruses as revealed in negatively stained preparations (top row), in thin-sectioned cells (middle row), and as compared with schematic diagrams (bottom row) (G. D. Hsiung et al., *Prog. Med. Virology* 25: 155, 1979).

DNA VIRUSES

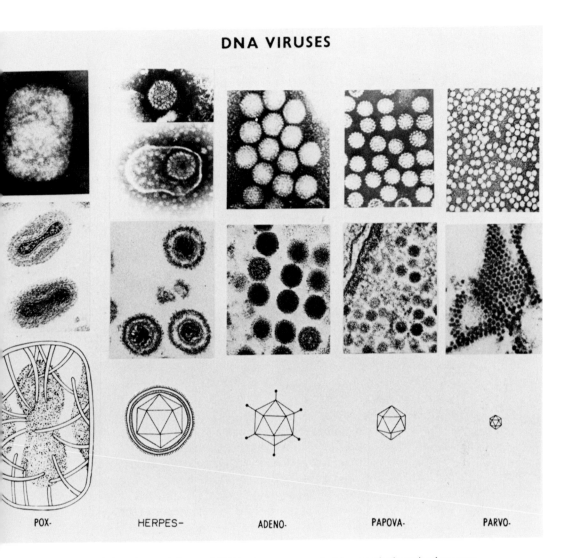

POX-   HERPES-   ADENO-   PAPOVA-   PARVO-

Figure 15. Relative size and shape of DNA viruses as revealed in negatively stained preparations (top row), in thin-sectioned cells (middle row), and as compared with schematic diagrams (bottom row) (G. D. Hsiung et al., *Prog. Med. Virology* 25: 154, 1979).

ferred to references cited at the end of part 2 (p. 85). For the purpose of rapid diagnosis, the procedures can be shortened from several days to several hours.

The procedures routinely used for fixation and embedding in the author's laboratory are:

1. *Primary fixation*. Fix tissue culture cells *in situ* with 2% glutaraldehyde in 0.1M cacodylate buffer, pH 7.2, or tissue fragments with a 3% glutaraldehyde solution in the same buffer. Tissue culture cells are fixed in monolayers *in situ* for 1 hour at 4°C, scraped, and then pelleted under low-speed centrifugation. Tissue blocks or fragments must be trimmed to a small size (1 mm^3) for primary and post-fixation. All fixed specimens are washed in 3 changes of 0.1M cacodylate buffer containing 0.18M sucrose, and stored in the same buffer overnight at 4°C.

2. *Post-fixation*. Place the tissue blocks in 1.33% osmium-collidine fixative for 1 hour at 4°C (for formula, see below).

3. En bloc *staining*. Rinse specimens with triple-distilled water 3 times; stain *en bloc* with 0.5% uranyl acetate for 4 hours at 4°C.

4. *Dehydration*. Use the following concentrations of ethanol: 50%, 70%, 80%, 95%, and 100% (3 changes each).

5. *Penetration and infiltration*. Place specimens in propylene oxide for 15 minutes each for 2 changes, then in a 1:1 mixture of propylene oxide and Epon overnight at 4°C.

6. *Embedding*. Add freshly prepared Epon mixture to the specimens and let stand for 1 hour at room temperature. Transfer specimens to Epon-filled Beem capsules for polymerization at 60°C for 48 hours.

7. *Trimming block*. Cut off excess Epon at the tips of the blocks in order to reach specimens easily.

8. *Sectioning*. Thin sectioning is the most tedious step and requires considerable experience. The two ultramicrotomes most widely used are the Sorvall and the LKB. Microtomes from other sources such as Leitz, Reichert and Cambridge are also satisfactory. Glass knives can be used but diamond knives originally described by Fernandez-Moran are superior and nearly essential for sectioning Epon 812. The thickness of the sections can be accurately judged from the interference colors, ranging from bright colors for fairly thick sections to dull grays for the very thin ones (gray: <600Å; silver: 600–900Å). Sections are placed on grids for staining and examination.

9. *Staining*. (a) Add a drop of uranyl acetate staining solution (0.5%) to a petri dish with wax on the bottom; place the grid with sections down on the staining solution for approximately 10–12 minutes and then rinse 3 times in distilled water. (The length of time required for staining varies depending on tissue specimen and embedding media.) (b) Place a drop of lead citrate staining solution in a petri dish with wax on the bottom. (Add a small weighing dish containing a few pellets of NaOH to the petri dish to absorb CO_2 in the air and to prevent precipitation of the

lead salt solution during staining.) Place the grids with sections down over the staining solution for 10–12 minutes, rinse first in 0.02N NaOH, then in distilled water.

10. *EM examination.* The doubly stained sections are ready for EM examination. Figures 14 and 15 illustrate the relative size and shape of major groups of viruses that infect humans as revealed in negatively stained preparations and in thin-sectioned infected cells.

REAGENTS

0.2M Sodium Cacodylate

Weigh out 42.8 gm sodium cacodylate ($C_2H_6AsNaO_2 \cdot 3H_2O$) and add distilled water to make 1000 ml. Adjust pH to 7.3.

0.1M Sodium Cacodylate–0.18M Sucrose (Buffer Washing Solution)

0.2M Cacodylate	250 ml
Sucrose	30.8 gm

Add distilled water to make 500 ml. Adjust pH to 7.3.

2% Glutaraldehyde–0.1M Sodium Cacodylate

0.2M Sodium Cacodylate	300 ml
50% Glutaraldehyde	24 ml

Add distilled water to make 600 ml. Adjust pH to 7.3.

3% Glutaraldehyde–0.1M Sodium Cacodylate

0.2M Sodium Cacodylate	300 ml
50% Glutaraldehyde	36 ml

Add distilled water to make 600 ml. Adjust pH to 7.3.

Osmium-Collidine Fixative (Bennet & Luft, 1959)

2% OsO_4	6.7 ml
0.2M s-collidine buffer, pH 7.4 (2,4,6-trimethylpyridine)	3.3 ml

The final pH should be 7.4.

Epon Mixture (Luft)

1. *Mixture A*

Epon 812	62 ml
Dodecenyl succinic anhydride	100 ml

2. *Mixture B*

Epon 812	100 ml
Nadic methyl anhydride	89 ml

Mixtures A and B are made in advance and stored separately at −20°C. Before use, warm to room temperature and mix A to B in the proportion of

4:6; add 0.15 ml DMP (2,4,6-tri(dimethylaminomethyl) phenol) per 10 ml of the final mixture.

Uranyl Acetate Solution

Uranyl acetate solution is made either 0.5% in distilled water or 10% in 25% ethanol. The solutions are filtered by millipore-membrane ultrafiltration and stored in a tightly capped tube at room temperature away from light.

Lead Citrate Solution

Weigh out 30–35 mg lead citrate and add to 10 ml distilled water. Shake intermittently for 30 minutes. Add drops of 5N NaOH and shake vigorously until mixture is clear. Centrifuge for 15 minutes before use. This solution should be stored in a tightly stoppered tube and clarified by centrifugation each time before use.

11. Physicochemical Methods for Characterization of Major Virus Groups

Many systems have been proposed for the classification of viruses, but there is general agreement that physical and chemical properties, such as nucleic acid type, size, and structure of a virus, are the basic characteristics on which to base a taxonomic scheme. Table 11 lists some of the major characteristics of selected animal viruses infecting humans.

Methods for determining nucleic acid types, size, shape, and lipid content of each virus family are described only briefly below. Detailed descriptions of each virus group and certain virus types within the groups are discussed separately in the following chapters.

It should be pointed out that physical and chemical methods are not routinely used in a diagnostic laboratory. However, there are instances when newly isolated viruses cannot be identified by standard serologic techniques. In such situations it may be necessary to study the agent's more basic properties, including nucleic acid type (RNA or DNA), size, shape, and ether-sensitivity, in order to characterize it taxonomically. The procedures described below are applicable to a small clinical virology laboratory setting.

NUCLEIC ACID DETERMINATION

The nucleic acid type can be determined by a number of methods. The most common method is based on the ability of certain compounds, such as 5-bromo-2-deoxyuridine (BUDR), to inhibit the multiplication of DNA viruses but not affect the multiplication of RNA viruses. Thus, in a cell culture containing BUDR at a concentration of 40 µg per ml, CPE induced by herpes simplex virus (a DNA virus) is completely inhibited, whereas CPE induced by an enterovirus (an RNA virus) is not affected.

It should be noted that the inhibitory effect of the drug is greater in passaged cell lines than in primary monkey kidney cell cultures; furthermore, cer-

Table 11. Physicochemical Characteristics of Viruses Infecting Humans

Nucleic Acid Type	Symmetry of Nucleocapsid	Virion[a]	Size (nm)	Virus Family[b]	Viruses Encountered in a Clinical Laboratory
RNA	icosahedral	N	25 – 30	picornaviridae	poliovirus coxsackievirus echovirus rhinovirus
	icosahedral	E	40 – 70	togaviridae	alphavirus flavivirus
	icosahedral	E	60	rubiviridae	rubella virus
	icosahedral	N	70 – 80	reoviridae	reovirus rotavirus
	helical	E	80 – 120	myxoviridae	influenza virus
	helical	E	150 – 300	paramyxoviridae	parainfluenza virus mumps virus
	helical	E	150 – 300	pseudomyxoviridae	measles viruses RSV
	helical	E	60 × 180	rhabdoviridae	rabies virus
DNA	icosahedral	N	45 – 55	papovaviridae	wart, BK, JC virus
	icosahedral	N	70 – 80	adenoviridae	adenovirus
	icosahedral	E	150 – 200	herpesviridae	herpes simplex virus, cytomegalovirus, varicella-zoster virus, Epstein-Barr virus
	complex	E	230 × 300	poxviridae	vaccinia virus

[a]E = enveloped, sensitive to ether treatment; N = naked, resistant to ether treatment.

[b]Other viruses not listed in this table are: coronaviridae, arenaviridae, and retroviridae of the RNA type, measuring 80–160 nm, with helical nucleocapsids, each surrounded by an envelope; and parvoviridae, containing single-stranded DNA, 18–20 nm in diameter and having nucleocapsids without envelopes.

78

tain DNA viruses, including adenovirus and papovavirus, may not be affected by BUDR; use of other DNA inhibitors may be necessary.

1. Make serial 10-fold dilutions of an unknown virus suspension from 10^{-1} to 10^{-6}.
2. Inoculate each dilution into two sets of cell culture tubes: one set of cultures containing medium with an inhibitor, BUDR at 40 µg per ml; the other set to be used as a control, without the drug. Use two tubes per dilution and 0.1 ml inoculum per tube.
3. Compare virus infectivity titers in cultures with or without chemical inhibitors.
4. As controls, a known virus that is inhibited by BUDR as well as one that is not should be included in the test.

It is recognized that these procedures are indirect methods for nucleic acid determination. Therefore, interpretations of tests are tentative until more refined methods of nucleic acid extraction have been applied.

In selected instances, nucleic acid type can be determined by the use of acridine orange staining technique and/or Feulgen reaction. The appearance of a yellowish-green inclusion in the nucleus after acridine orange staining or a bright pink inclusion in a cell after Feulgen reaction is an indication that the nucleic acid of the virus is probably DNA. Electron microscopy, in addition to revealing viral structure, can also be used to determine nucleic acid type since DNA viruses generally stain intensely with uranyl acetate, whereas the RNA viruses do not.

These techniques, either individually or in combination, have been used for the determination of the nucleic acid of a variety of viruses.

SIZE AND STRUCTURE

Size and shape of a virus can be determined directly by electron microscopy when facilities are available. For example, direct electron microscopic examination of smears taken from lesions can be prepared within a few hours and the characteristic morphology of a virus can be observed and the size measured. Ultrathin sections of virus-infected cells also permit a direct approach to the determination of virus size, but distortion of the virus particle may occur during the process of fixation and dehydration.

The development of negative staining techniques with the use of electron-dense salts of phosphotungstic acid has permitted visualization of structural details, both surface and interior, of many virus types. However, when facilities are not available, the ultrafiltration method outlined below is useful for estimating the size of a virus particle.

Ultrafiltration is one of the simplest and oldest methods for measuring virus particle size. This is usually done by passing a virus suspension through a series of collodion membranes of graded porosity. The size of the virus is measured

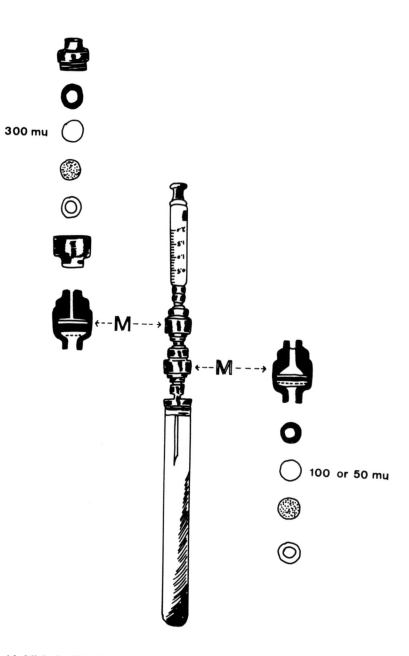

300 mµ

M

M

100 or 50 mµ

Figure 16. Mini-ultrafiltration equipment. Swinny adapter filter set.

    Teflon 0 ring gasket.

    Millipore membrane, 300, 100, or 50 nm.

    Supporting screen.

    Teflon flat gasket.

Table 12. Ultrafiltration for Estimating Virus Size[a]

Virus Size Range	Virus Infectivity (Limiting Pore Diameter of Millipore Membrane)	
	100 nm	50nm
Large	−	−
Medium	+	−
Small	+	+

[a]*Key*: virus infectivity detected after suspension passed through filter, +; virus infectivity not detected after suspension passed through filter. All suspensions are first passed through a 450- or 300-nm membrane in order to clarify the fluid.

grossly by its ability to pass through or be retained by the finest filter, although some limitations and complications have been encountered.

The availability of millipore filters and suitable holders has brought the ultrafiltration method within the scope of a small clinical laboratory. The equipment used for filtering small amounts of virus fluid is illustrated in figure 16. A 2-ml syringe is attached to two Swinny adaptors connected in series with a hypodermic needle and then sterilized. Either a Seitz membrane or a millipore membrane of 450- or 300-nm pore diameter is placed in the upper adaptor for clarifying virus fluid, and the test membrane of 100- or 50-nm diameter is placed in the lower adaptor. A 20-ml vacuum tube is used to collect the final filtrate. Millipore membranes of 300, 100 or 50 nm are sterilized by exposure to ultraviolet light for 10 minutes on each side. Virus infectivity of the suspension is determined before and after filtration; virus size is estimated according to the virus infectivity titers retained in the filtrates (table 12). Viruses of *large* size will not pass through 100-nm and 50-nm pore diameter membranes; therefore, the virus in a suspension that has lost its infectivity after passing through such membranes must be a large-size virus. The *medium*-size viruses pass through the 100-nm but not through 50-nm membranes; the *small* viruses pass through both 100- and 50-nm membranes.

1. Add 1–2 ml of unknown virus fluid into each of a series of filter sets containing 300-nm, 300- and 100-nm, and 300- and 50-nm filter membranes.
2. Make serial 10-fold dilutions from 10^{-1} to 10^{-6} of each filtrate as well as of the unfiltered virus suspension.
3. Inoculate each dilultion into a set of 2–4 culture tubes.
4. Compare virus infectivity titers of the unfiltered fluids with each of the filtrates. Estimate the size range of the unknown virus according to table 12.

LIPID CONTENT

Lipid content determination can be used to determine the presence of a lipid-containing envelope surrounding a virus. Diethyl ether, 20%–50% by volume, is added to an undiluted virus suspension; loss of virus infectivity is measured and those viruses that show no appreciable change in infectivity titer are considered ether-resistant. Chloroform or sodium deoxycholate (1:1000) can be used instead of ether in a similar manner to test for viral lipid content.

1. Add 0.5 ml of diethyl ether to 0.5 ml of an unknown virus suspension, shake vigorously, let stand at room temperature for 1–2 hours, and shake intermittently, or allow mixture to stand at 4°C for 18–24 hours.
2. Transfer the mixture into an open glass petri dish; allow the ether to evaporate.
3. Make serial 10-fold dilutions from 10^{-1} to 10^{-6} of both ether-treated and untreated virus suspensions.
4. Inoculate each dilution into a set of 2–4 culture tubes.
5. Compare virus infectivity titers of ether-treated and untreated samples.
6. As controls, known ether-sensitive and ether-resistant viruses should be included in the test.

ACID pH STABILITY TEST

Many viruses including the rhinovirus group are not stable at an acid pH. Thus a reduction in infectivity titers of 2–4 logs at pH 3.0 is an indication that the virus tested is an acid-labile one. The following test can be used:

1. To 5 ml of 0.2M tris buffer solution (pH 7.4), add drops of concentrated HCl in order to reach pH 3.0. Dilute the solution to a final volume of 20 ml with distilled water.
2. Add 0.2 ml of unknown virus suspension to 1.8 ml of the diluted buffer, pH 3.0. As a control, add 0.2 ml of the virus suspension to 1.8 ml of stock tris buffer, pH 7.4.
3. Keep the mixtures at room temperature for 3 hours.
4. Make serial 10-fold dilutions of the two mixtures and inoculate each into 2 or 3 culture tubes.
5. Compare virus infectivity titers of acid-treated and untreated samples.
6. Known acid-sensitive and acid-resistant viruses should be included in the test as additional controls.

Figure 17 schematically outlines the procedures described above and summarizes the physicochemical characteristics of the RNA and DNA viruses of the major virus groups.

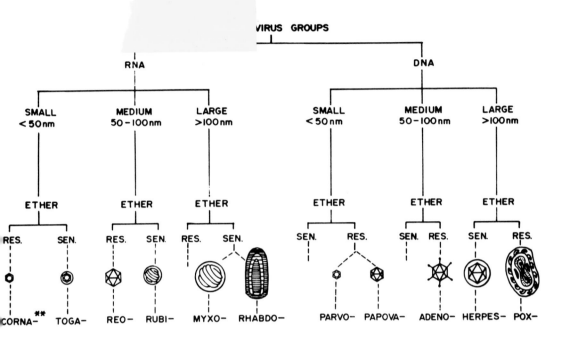

Figure 17. Major groups of viruses infecting humans: schematic diagram. RNA and DNA viruses are subdivided by size ranges: small, which pass through a 50-nm millipore filter; medium, which pass through a 100- but not a 50-nm filter; large, which do not pass through a 100-nm filter. RES. = resistant; SEN. = sensitive.

SUPPLEMENTARY READING FOR PART 2

Cell Culture for Virus Isolation and Assay

Clark, J., Schley, C., Irvine, K., and McIntosh, K. Comparison of cynomolgus and rhesus monkey kidney cells for recovery of viruses from clinical specimens. *J. Clin. Micro.* 9: 554, 1979.

Davis, P. M., and Phillpotts, R. J. Susceptibility of the Vero line of African green monkey kidney cells to human enteroviruses. *J. Hyg.* 72: 23, 1974.

Friedman, H. M., and Koropchak, C. Comparison of WI-38, MRC-5 and IMR-90 cell strains for isolation of viruses from clinical specimens. *J. Clin. Micro.* 7: 368, 1978.

Hollick, G. E., Reichrath, L., and Smith, T. F. Comparison of primary rhesus and cynomolgus monkey kidney culture for viral isolation from clinical specimens. *Am. J. Clin. Path.* 68: 276, 1977.

Howell, C. L., Miller, M. J., and Martin, W ⸺⸺⸺⸺⸺ rates of virus isolation
from leucocyte populations separated from ⸺⸺⸺⸺ ional and Ficoll-Paque/
Macrodex methods. *J. Clin. Micro.* 10: 533, 1979.

Hsiung, G. D. Applications of primary cell cultures in the study of animal viruses. III.
Biological and genetic studies of enteric viruses of man (enteroviruses). *Yale J. Biol.
Med.* 33: 359, 1961.

Landry, M. L., Mayo, D., and Hsiung, G. D. Comparison of guinea pig embryo cells,
rabbit kidney cells, and human embryonic lung fibroblast cell strains for isolation of
herpes simplex virus. *J. Clin. Micro.* 15: 842, 1982.

McSwiggan, D., Dorongar, S., Rahman, A. F., and Gibson, J. A. Comparison of the
sensitivity of human embryo kidney, HeLa cells, and WI-38 cells for the primary
isolation of viruses from the eye. *J. Clin. Pathol.* 28: 410, 1975.

Meguro, H., Bryant, J. D., Torrence, A. E., and Wright, P. F. Canine kidney cell
line for isolation of respiratory viruses. *J. Clin. Micro.* 9: 175, 1979.

Reed, L. J., and Muench, H. A simple method for estimating fifty percent endpoints.
Am. J. Hyg. 27: 493, 1938.

Schmidt, N. J., Ho, H. H., Riggs, J. L., and Lennette, E. H. Comparative sensitivity of
various cell culture systems for isolation of viruses from waste water and fecal samples. *Appl. Environ. Micro.* 36: 480, 1978.

Enzyme-Linked Immunosorbent Assay

Harmon, M. W., Drake, S., and Kasel, J. A. Detection of adenovirus by enzyme-
linked immunosorbent assay. *J. Clin. Micro.* 9: 342, 1979.

Voller, B. A., and Bidwell, D. E. Bacteria microplate enzyme immunoassay system for
measurement of cytomegalovirus. *J. Clin. Micro.* 11: 546, 1980.

Voller, B. A., Bidwell, D. E., and Bartlett, A. Microplate enzyme immunoassays for
the immunodiagnosis of viral infection. In *Manual of clinical immunology*, ed. N. R.
Rose and H. Friedman, p. 506. Washington, D. C.: American Society for Microbiology, 1976.

Yolken, R. H. Enzyme-linked immunosorbent assay (ELISA): a practical tool for rapid
diagnosis of viruses and other infectious agents. *Yale J. Biol. Med.* 53: 85, 1980.

Yolken, R. H., Kim, H. W., Clem, T., Wyatt, R. G., Kalica, A. R., Chanock, R. M.,
and Kapikian, A. Z. Enzyme-linked immunosorbent assay (ELISA) for detection of
human reovirus-like agent of infantile gastroenteritis. *Lancet* 2: 263, 1977.

Yolken, R. H., and Stopa, P. J. Comparison of seven enzyme immunoassay systems for
measurement of cytomegalovirus. *J. Clin. Micro.* 11: 546, 1980.

Acridine Orange Staining

Gluck, L., and Kulovich, M. V. Histochemical studies of the distribution of RNA in
tissues of the developing chick embryo. *Yale J. Biol. Med.* 36: 379, 1964.

Mayor, H. D., and Melnick, J. L. Intracellular and extracellular reactions of viruses
with vital dyes. *Yale J. Biol. Med.* 34: 340, 1961.

Immunofluorescent Staining Techniques

Gardner, P. S., and McQuillin, J. *Rapid virus diagnosis: application of immunofluorescence.* Toronto: Butterworth and Co., Ltd., 1974.

Lyerla, H. C., and Forrester, F. T. *Immunofluorescence methods in virology*. Washington, D. C.: U.S. Dept. of HEW, Public Health Service, 1979.

Immunoperoxidase Test

Avrameas, S., and Ternynck, T. Peroxidase labeled antibody and Fab conjugates with enhanced intracellular penetration. *Immunochemistry* 8: 1175, 1971.

Forghani, B., Schmidt, N. J., and Dennis, J. Antibody assays for varicella-zoster virus: comparison of enzyme immunoassay with neutralization, immune adherence hemagglutination, and complement fixation. *J. Clin. Micro.* 8: 545, 1978.

Gardner, P. S., Grandieu, M., and McQuillin, J. Comparison of immunofluorescence and immunoperoxidase methods for viral diagnosis at a distance. A WHO Collaborative Study. *Bull. W.H.O.* 56: 105, 1978.

Graham, R. C., Jr., and Karnovsky, M. J. The early stages of absorption of injected horseradish peroxidase in the proximal tubules of mouse kidney: ultrastructural cytochemistry by a new technique. *J. Histochem. Cytochem.* 14: 291, 1966.

Nakane, P. K., and Pierce, G. B. Enzyme-labeled antibodies: preparation and application for localization of antigens. *J. Histochem. Cytochem.* 14: 929, 1966.

Sternberger, L. A., Hardy, P. H., Jr., Cuculis, J. J., and Meyer, H. G. The unlabeled antibody enzyme method of immunohistochemistry. Preparation and properties of soluble antigen-antibody complex (horseradish peroxidase) and its use in identification of spirochetes. *J. Histochem. Cytochem.* 18: 315, 1970.

Electron Microscopy

Books and Review Papers

Almeida, J. D. Practical aspects of diagnostic electron microscopy. *Yale J. Biol. Med.* 53: 5, 1980.

Almeida, J. D., and Waterson, A. P. The morphology of virus-antibody interaction. *Adv. Virus Res.* 5: 307, 1969.

Dalton, A. J., and Haguenan, F. *Ultrastructure of animal viruses and bacteriophages: an atlas*. New York: Academic Press, 1973.

Doane, F. W. Virus morphology as an aid for rapid diagnosis. *Yale J. Biol. Med.* 53: 19, 1980.

Doane, F. W. Identification of viruses by immuno-electron microscopy. In *Viral immunodiagnosis*, ed. E. Kurstak and R. Morisset, p. 237. New York: Academic Press, 1974.

Horne, R. W., and Wildy, P. Virus structure revealed by negative staining. *Adv. Virus Res.* 10: 101, 1963.

Hsiung, G. D., Fong, C. K. Y., and August, M. J. The use of electron microscopy in diagnosis of viral infection. *Prog. Med. Virol.* 25: 133, 1979.

Specific Articles

Anderson, N., and Doane, F. W. Agar diffusion method for negative staining of microbial suspensions in salt solutions. *Appl. Microbiol.* 24: 495, 1972.

Bennett, H. S., and Leift, J. H. S-collidine as a basis for buffering fixatives. *J. Biophys. Biochem. Cytol.* 6: 113, 1959.

Doane, F. W., Anderson, N., Chao, J., and Noonan, A. Two hour embedding procedure for intracellular detection of viruses by electron microscopy. *Appl. Microbiol.* 27: 407, 1974.

Frasca, J. M., and Parks, V. R. A routine technique for double-staining ultrathin sections using uranyl and lead salts. *J. Cell Biol.* 25: 157, 1965.

Hammond, G. W., Hazelton, P. R., Chuang, I., and Klisko, B. Improved detection of viruses by electron microscopy after direct ultracentrifuge preparation of specimens. *J. Clin. Micro.* 14: 210, 1981.

Luft, J. M. Improvements in epoxy resin embedding methods. *J. Biophys. Biochem. Cytol.* 9: 409, 1961.

Reynolds, E. S. The use of lead citrate at high pH as an electron-opaque stain in electron microscopy. *J. Cell Biol.* 17: 208, 1963.

Sabatini, D. D., Bensch, K., and Barrnett, R. J. Cytochemistry and electron microscopy. The preservation of cellular ultrastructure and enzymatic activity by aldehyde fixation. *J. Cell Biol.* 17: 19, 1963.

New Developments in Immunologic Tests

McIntosh, K., Wilfert, C., Chernesky, M., and Mattheis, M. J. Summary of a workshop on new and useful methods in rapid viral diagnosis. *J. Infect. Dis.* 142: 793, 1980.

McIntosh, K., Wilfert, C., Chernesky, M., Plotkin, S., and Mattheis, M. J. Summary of a workshop on new and useful methods in viral diagnosis. *J. Infect. Dis.* 138: 414, 1978.

PART 3: Recognition and Characterization of Viruses by Virus Morphology and Virus-Induced Cellular Changes

RNA VIRUSES

12. Picornaviridae

Picornaviridae includes the enteroviruses and the rhinoviruses (table 13). The name was adopted by the International Committee on Taxonomy of Viruses as a derivation of "pico," meaning very small, and "RNA," the nucleic acid type present in all members of the group.

ENTEROVIRUSES

The enteroviruses include 3 types of poliovirus, 24 types of coxsackie A, 6 types of coxsackie B, and some 34 types of echovirus or enteric cytopathogenic human orphan virus. Starting with enterovirus type 68, all enteroviruses will be designated numerically. The human alimentary tract is the natural habitat for these viruses. They can be recovered from patients with a variety of illnesses, including poliomyelitis, aseptic meningitis, myocarditis, and pericarditis. In addition to their pathogenicity in humans, the polioviruses produce paralysis in monkeys. The coxsackieviruses are highly pathogenic for newborn mice, but the echovirus group rarely induces disease in experimental animals.

Morphologically, all enteroviruses, whether in infected cells or in infected tissues, are similar (figures 18 and 19). They are small, 25 to 30 nm, have icosahedral symmetry, with 32 capsomeres, and contain a single-stranded RNA core. Viruses in this group are relatively stable at pH 3.0 and are ether-resistant. Storage at $-20°C$ is satisfactory for several years.

The discovery by Enders et al. in 1949 that poliovirus can be propagated in cell culture of non–nerve tissue origin greatly facilitated the diagnosis and ultimate control of poliomyelitis and other enterovirus infections. Most enteroviruses propagate readily only in cell cultures of primate origin, although certain types of coxsackie A virus can replicate in guinea pig embryo (GPE) cell cultures. Furthermore, the susceptibility of various species of monkey kidney cell cultures to these viruses has been found to differ.

Table 13. Host Cell Susceptibility and Pathogenicity of Human Enteroviruses and Rhinoviruses

| Virus Type | Serotypes | Acid Stability (pH 3.0) | Primary Cell Culture | | | Passaged Cell Line | | | | Hemagglutination[a] |
			HEK	RhMK or GMK	RK/GPE	HDF	Hep-2 Hela	Vero	Newborn Mice	
Enterovirus										
Poliovirus	1–3	stable	++	++	–	++	++	++	–	–
Coxsackie virus B	1–6		++	++	–	++	++	++	++	+/–
Coxsackie virus A	1–24[a]		+/–	+/–	–/+	–	–	–	++	+/–
Echovirus	1–34[b]		+	++	–	+	–	–	–	+/–
Enterovirus	68–71[c]		+	++	e	+	–	–	–	
Rhinovirus	1–89	labile	+/–	+/–	–	++	+/–	–	–	–

[a] Coxsackievirus A13 cross reacts with coxsackievirus A18.
[b] Echovirus 1 cross reacts with echovirus 8; echovirus 9 cross reacts with coxsackievirus A23; echovirus 10 reclassified as reovirus type 1.
[c] Enterovirus starting with type 68 will be designated numerically.
[d] Coxsackievirus B-1, 3, 5, and echovirus 6, 7, 12, 20, 21, 24, 29, 30 and 33 hemagglutinate human type-O cells at 37°C. Coxsackie virus A-20, 21, 24, and echovirus 3, 11, 13, and 19 hemagglutinate human type-O cells at 4°C.
[e] Test not done.

Key: + = virus-induced change
    – = no change

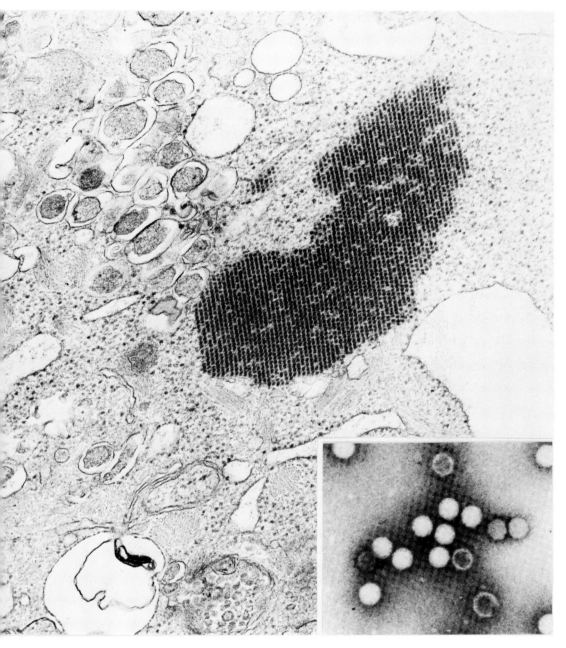

Figure 18. Electron micrograph of poliovirus type 1 in an infected Hep-2 cell. A large aggregate of virus particles in crystalline arrays is present in the cytoplasm (48,000X). Inset: Poliovirus particles stained with PTA (168,000X).

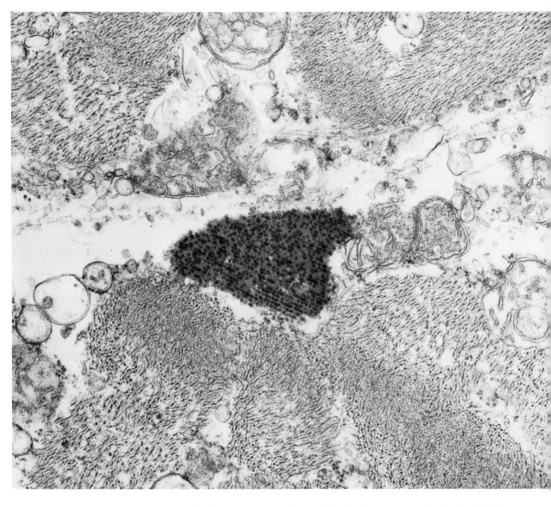

Figure 19. Electron micrograph of an aggregate of coxsackie A-10 virus particles in the hind-leg skeletal muscle cell of an infected mouse (38,400X).

Among the primate cell cultures, rhesus and cynomolgus or African green monkey kidney cells are highly sensitive to virtually all enteroviruses; cell cultures from other African monkeys, for example the patas monkey (*Erythrocebus patas*), are only susceptible to certain ones; the New World monkey kidney cells are generally resistant. Human kidney cultures seem to be the most suitable system for isolation of the echoviruses. Except for certain types of coxsackie A viruses, nonprimate cell cultures are generally resistant to infection by human enteroviruses. Certain passaged cell strains, including human embryo fibroblast cells, WI-38 cells and other types, are currently being used with success for enterovirus isolation and are readily available commercially. All coxsackieviruses are also pathogenic to newborn mice, which provide the most uniform and sensitive system for isolation of this group of viruses.

Specimen Inoculation

Stool or rectal swabs are the specimens of choice for isolation of enteroviruses; cerebrospinal fluids and/or throat swabs can also be used. Suitable tissue culture types for inoculation of specimens include primary monkey kidney cells and/or human cell lines. These consist of rhesus monkey kidney (RhMK) or African green monkey kidney (GMK), human diploid fibroblast (HDF), WI-38, human embryonic kidney (HEK) and/or Hep-2 cell lines, depending upon what is available. If, however, coxsackie A viruses are suspected, specimens should be inoculated either directly into newborn mice or into guinea pig embryo (GPE) cells, if available.

Virus Isolation, Propagation, and Assay

Cytopathic effect in fluid cultures. Observation for cytopathic effect (CPE) is the most sensitive and rapid method for recognition of enterovirus infection in cell culture. Examples of the typical CPE induced by poliovirus type 1 in RhMK and Hep-2 cells are shown in figure 20. Extensive cell destruction usually occurs 24 to 48 hours after inoculation into either cell system. However, CPE induced by echoviruses is selectively dependent upon the type of cell culture used. Examples indicating the differences in sensitivity of the three cell systems are shown in figures 20 and 21, where echovirus 11 induced extensive CPE in human kidney cell cultures within a few hours of inoculation; only small areas of degeneration in rhesus monkey kidney cultures (figure 21); and no CPE in Hep-2 cells (figure 20). Certain group A coxsackieviruses induce distinctive CPE in GPE cells (figure 22), a useful new diagnostic tool when GPE cells are available.

Mouse pathogenicity. Newborn mice infected with coxsackieviruses show illness 4 to 7 days after inoculation. Hind limb paralysis is usually observed in mice inoculated with coxsackie A-9 (figure 23) 4 days after inoculation; death occurs in 5 to 7 days. The coxsackieviruses can be subdivided into groups A and B, determined by histological lesions produced in mice; group A coxsackie-

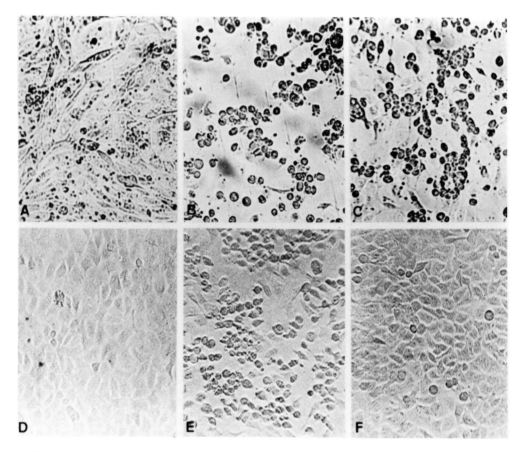

Figure 20. Cytopathic effect (CPE) induced by poliovirus type 1 and echovirus type 11 in RhMK and Hep-2 cultures (100X).

A. Uninoculated RhMK culture.

B. CPE induced by poliovirus type 1 in RhMK culture, 1 day after inoculation.

C. CPE induced by echovirus type 11 in RhMK culture, 4 days after inoculation.

D. Uninoculated Hep-2 culture.

E. CPE induced by poliovirus type 1 in Hep-2 culture, 1 day after inoculation.

F. Absence of CPE in Hep-2 culture infected with echovirus type 11, 4 days after inoculation.

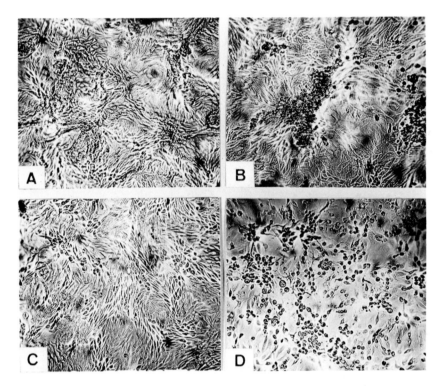

Figure 21. Cytopathic effect induced by echovirus type 11, WB strain, in RhMK and HEK cultures (100X) (G. D. Hsiung, *Yale J. Biol. Med.* 33: 359, 1961).

A. Uninoculated RhMK culture.

B. CPE induced by echovirus type 11 in RhMK culture, 2 days after infection, showing small foci of degeneration.

C. Uninoculated HEK culture.

D. CPE induced by echovirus type 11, 8 hours after infection, showing extensive cellular degeneration.

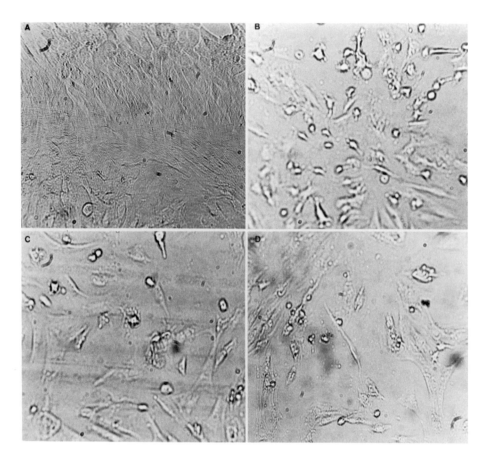

Figure 22. Cytopathic effect induced by group A coxsackieviruses in GPE cell cultures (100X) (modified from Landry et al., *Clinical Micro*. 13: 588, 1981).
    A. Uninoculated GPE culture.
    B. Coxsackievirus type A-10, 2 days after inoculation.
    C. Coxsackievirus type A-2, 3 days after inoculation.
    D. Coxsackievirus type A-5, 3 days after inoculation.

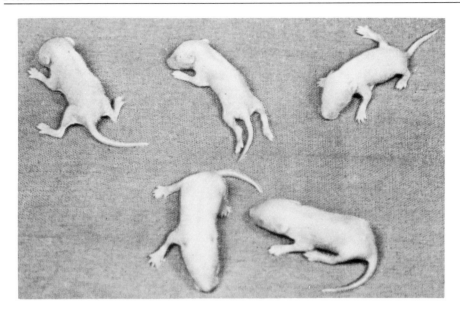

Figure 23. Paralysis induced by coxsackievirus type A-9 in suckling mice, four days after intraperitoneal inoculation; the mouse in the center (top) showed severe paralysis of hind
legs (R. H. A. Swain and T. C. Dodds, *Clinical virology*, Edinburgh: Livingstone,
1967, p. 175).

viruses cause generalized myositis, whereas group B coxsackieviruses cause
focal myositis, especially in heart muscle.

Plaque formation in bottle cultures. Monolayer cell cultures infected with certain members of the enterovirus group exhibit plaque formation under agar overlay medium. Plaques are colorless areas of dead cells surrounded by viable
cells, which are stained with neutral red, a vital dye. Different enterovirus types
induce plaques of varying size and shape (figure 24), in much the same manner
that different bacteria produce characteristic colonies on agar plates. Poliovirus
plaques are large and clear; coxsackievirus plaques are of medium size and have
hazy centers. With the exception of echovirus type 7, most of the echovirus
plaques are small and irregular. Selective differences in cell susceptibility are
also illustrated under agar overlay. Echovirus type 11 induces large, clear
plaques with high virus titers in HEK cells but small, irregular plaques in the
RhMK culture (figure 25). Poliovirus type 1 induces large clear plaques in both
rhesus and patas monkey kidney (patas MK) cells, whereas echovirus type 1
produces plaques in the RhMK but not in the patas MK culture (figure 26). Thus
the plaque method in adjunct with selective cell susceptibility is a useful tool
for the recognition and separation of mixed virus infections. Theoretically one
infectious virus particle initiates a single plaque; thus pure virus stock can be
obtained by picking a single plaque and subculturing it into the same host system. In addition, virus plaque counts are accurate quantitative assay methods
for determining virus infectivity titers.

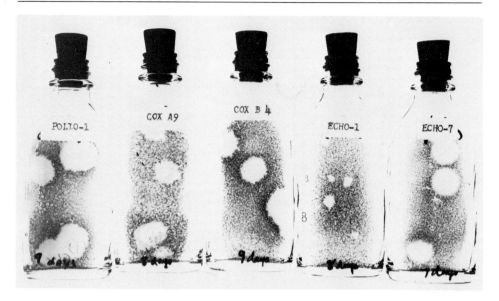

Figure 24. Plaque morphology of different enteroviruses in RhMK cultures. Left to right: Polio-
virus type 1 (Mahoney), coxsackievirus type A-9 (Grigg), coxsackievirus type B-4
(Texas 13), echovirus type 1 (Farouk), and echovirus type 7 (Garnett) (G. D. Hsiung,
Yale J. Biol. Med. 33: 359, 1961).

Identification of Isolates

Neutralization test. Identifying enteroviruses by serological means is becoming
a difficult task because of the increasing number of virus types in this group.
Neutralization tests in tissue culture (see p. 29) using serum pools is one means
of facilitating the typing of enteroviruses. The intersecting serum scheme in-
volves a number of combinations of antisera, each serum being represented in
two pools; the identity of the virus type is indicated by the serum type neutralizing the agent present in the two pools sharing a common component. The use
of serum pools has proven to be a relatively rapid and satisfactory technique for
identifying enteroviruses, although the neutralization test procedure is still rather
laborious and time-consuming. In addition, the method does not provide information for ready recognition of mixed virus types.

Cell culture selectivity. A simple diagnostic tool is urgently needed for rapid
typing within the enterovirus group, which includes some 71 serotypes, and
probably more that will be discovered. Advantage can be taken of the differences
in susceptibility of host cell systems, mouse pathogenicity, and rate of appearance of enterovirus CPE for preliminary diagnosis of these viruses; a presumptive diagnosis can be made as soon as typical CPE appears in certain cell culture types. Thus, many serum pools can be eliminated and serologic testing can
be simplified. Final identification, however, of a virus type within the group can
only be made by neutralization test using type-specific antiserum. It should be

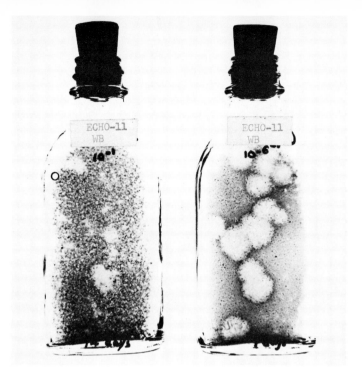

Figure 25. Plaque formation of echovirus type 11, WB strain, in RhMK and HEK cultures. Left: RhMK inoculated with 0.1 ml of 10^{-1} dilution of virus, showing small irregular plaques. Right: HEK culture inoculated with 10^{-6} dilution of the same virus suspension, showing large circular plaques.

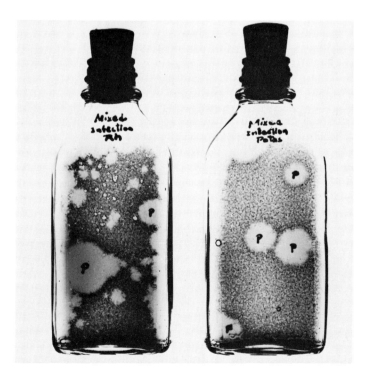

Figure 26. Mixed infection with two enteroviruses: monkey kidney cultures inoculated with a fecal specimen containing two different enteroviruses. Left: Rhesus monkey kidney culture showing both poliovirus type 1 (large circular plaques) and echovirus type 1 (small irregular plaques). Right: Patas monkey kidney culture showing only poliovirus plaques (G. D. Hsiung and D. M. Horstmann, *Conn. Med.* 25: 403, 1961).

noted that some difficulties may be encountered when serial cell lines are used, since susceptibility to a given virus type may be inconsistent as a result of differences in cell sublines carried by various laboratories.

Electron microscopy is not generally used to diagnose enterovirus infections. However, rapid identification of an isolate as an enterovirus can be made by negative staining of a suspension of the virus isolate grown in cell culture. Enterovirus particles also can be identified by size and shape in thin sections of virus-infected cells. This is illustrated by the presence of virus aggregates forming a characteristic crystalline array in the cytoplasm of infected cells (figures 18 and 19). Since group A coxsackieviruses do not grow readily in cell culture, the visualization by EM of typical virus particles in tissue specimens, such as skeletal muscle of infected mice (figure 19), has provided the basis for efforts to utilize electron microscopy as a means to detect and identify the presence of virus particles in tissues suspected of harboring virus from this group.

Serodiagnosis

A number of methods have been employed in the serologic diagnosis of enterovirus infection. However, diagnosis of enterovirus infections by serological tests is not routinely attempted except in selected cases when infection with one of a few specific enterovirus types is suspected. In this instance, the neutralization test in cell cultures is usually applied with acute and convalescent sera for antibody rises.

Special Markers for Differentiation of Virulent and Attenuated Poliovirus Isolates in Cell Culture

Certain *in vitro* tests that measure poliovirus's sensitivity to concentration of bicarbonate, incubation temperature, and rate of neutralization have been used for determining virus virulence. Only the first two markers mentioned will be discussed in this section.

The D marker refers to differences in sensitivity of poliovirus strains to low bicarbonate concentrations in the agar overlay medium. In attenuated strains (classified as $D-$) the appearance of plaques is delayed or inhibited, whereas in virulent strains ($D+$) plaque formation proceeds equally well in low as in high bicarbonate concentrations. The $T_{40°C}$ markers refers to the ability of virulent strains ($T+$) to grow at 40°C; attentuated strains ($T-$) show a marked reduction in titer (4 to 5 logs) at this temperature when compared to titers obtained when incubation is carried out at 36°C. Tests for the $T_{40°C}$ marker can be carried out by either the CPE or the plaque method, but only the plaque method is used for the D marker. The $T_{40°C}$ incubation temperature is critical; it should not go below 39°C nor above 40°C during the 4

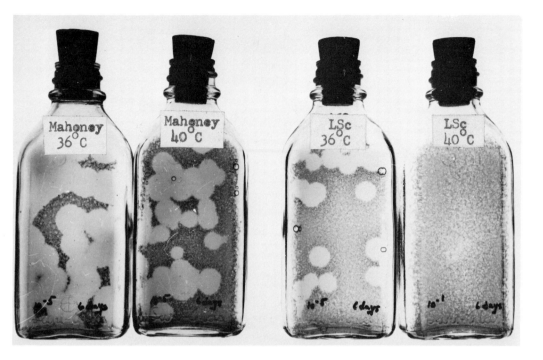

Figure 27. Differentiation of virulent and attenuated poliovirus type 1, determined by varying the incubation temperature (T marker). Two bottles at left: Virulent poliovirus (Mahoney) incubated at 36°C and 40°C respectively. Two bottles at right: Attenuated poliovirus (LSc) incubated at 36°C and 40°C respectively; note absence of plaques at 40°C.

days of incubation. The results of a T-marker test by the plaque method are illustrated in figure 27.

1. Make serial 10-fold dilutions from 10^{-1} to 10^{-6} of poliovirus suspension and inoculate each into two sets of bottle cultures.
2. T markers: overlay with the regular agar overlay medium (overlay medium, see p. 32) and incubate one set at 35°C–36°C and the other set at 39°C–40°C. Terminate incubation at 4 days and count the number of plaque-forming units (PFUs).
3. D markers: overlay one set of bottle cultures with high and the other set with low concentrations of $NaHCO_3$ in the media (for preparation of media, see p. 32) and incubate at 37°C. Terminate incubation at 4 days and count the PFUs.
4. Calculate T and D efficiency of plating (EOP) as follows (see also figure 27):

Example: T markers for Poliovirus Type 1

Incubation Temperature	Virus titers, PFUs per 0.1 ml	
	Mahoney (virulent)	LSc (attenuated)
40°C	1.3×10^7	10^1
36°C	2.4×10^7	1.1×10^6

$$\text{EOP} = \frac{1.3 \times 10^7}{2.4 \times 10^7} = 0.5 \quad \text{EOP} = \frac{10^1}{1.1 \times 10^6} = 0.000009$$

Example: D markers for poliovirus type 1

Overlay Medium	Virus titers, PFU per 0.1 ml	
	Mahoney (virulent)	LSc (attenuated)
Low $NaHCO_3$	1.9×10^7	10^1
High $NaHCO_3$	2.4×10^7	1×10^6

$$\text{EOP} = \frac{1.9 \times 10^7}{2.4 \times 10^7} = 0.5 \quad \text{EOP} = \frac{10^1}{1 \times 10^6} = 0.00001$$

5. When EOP is equal to or greater than 0.1, the virus strain is considered virulent, whereas an EOP equal to 0.00001 or less is considered an avirulent strain; intermediate strains have EOP values in between.

RHINOVIRUSES

The rhinovirus group consists of some 113 types, with 89 established serotypes known principally as the causative agents of the common cold. Man is their natural host, and no laboratory animal has yet been found susceptible to infection. Rhinoviruses can be isolated from the nose and throat but not from the feces of patients with acute afebrile upper-respiratory disease.

The physical and chemical as well as morphological properties of the rhinoviruses are similar to those of the enteroviruses except that the rhinoviruses are unstable at acid pH (pH 3.0). Growth of rhinovirus generally is facilitated by incubation at 33°C in rotating culture tubes containing media at neutral pH, conditions similar to those of the mucous membranes of the nasal cavities.

The tissue cultures are the only known system for propagation of the rhinoviruses. Based on cell selectivity, the rhinoviruses have been subdivided into the H strain and the M strain. The H viruses propagate best in human cells, both primary cultures and diploid cell strains such as WI-38 and others; the M viruses produce cytopathic effect in primary rhesus monkey as well as in human cells, including some of the continuous cell lines such as those derived from carcinoma of human nasopharynx (KB) and of human cervix (HeLa). However, since the ability of rhinoviruses to replicate in monkey cells is variable, this method is not commonly used for differentiation.

Specimen Inoculation

Nasal washings or nasal swabs and throat swabs should be inoculated directly into cultures immediately after collection, without freezing if possible. Human diploid cell strains, human embryonic kidney, or other primary human fibroblast cells are satisfactory. All cultures should be maintained at a neutral pH and incubated at 33°C in a roller drum, if available.

Virus Isolation, Propagation, and Assay

Cytopathic effect in fluid cultures. The CPE induced by rhinovirus in human diploid cell strain, WI-38, and in HeLa cell culture is shown in figures 28 and 29. These cellular changes resemble those of an enterovirus but develop rather slowly upon primary isolation. Under favorable conditions, that is, in culture tubes maintained at pH 6.8–7.0 and incubated at 33°C in a roller drum, rhinovirus-induced CPE generally appears within 2 weeks.

Plaque formation in bottle cultures. Rhinoviruses induce plaques in HeLa cell cultures under starch gel or agar overlay media. Examples are shown in figure 30. Different strains of rhinovirus produce various sizes of large, intermediate, and small plaques.

Growth in organ culture. Isolation of certain rhinovirus types can be facilitated by using organ cultures of human embryonic trachea. As illustrated in figure 31, the decreasing ciliary activity and the progressive degenerative changes in an organ culture indicate the presence of a rhinovirus. The following procedure is used for the preparation of a human trachea culture:

1. Place freshly collected trachea tissue in a medium containing Hanks' BSS with 10% fetal bovine serum, and prepare for cultures as soon as possible.
2. Wash the trachea tissue in Hanks' BSS and cut into small pieces, 2–3 mm^2 in size.
3. Crosshatch 4–6 small patches on the bottom of a small plastic petri dish.
4. Place a small piece of the tissue, ciliated side up, on each patch (tissues will adhere to the scratched area).
5. Add nutrient consisting of Medium-199 with 0.35% $NaHCO_3$, 5 ml medium per 60-mm petri dish. (Specimen, 0.1–0.3 ml, can be inoculated into the dish with trachea tissue.)
6. Incubate the petri dish in 5% CO_2 mixed with 95% compressed air, at 33°C–35°C.
7. Examine ciliary activity under an inverted microscope at daily intervals.
8. Harvest culture fluid for virus identification when decreasing ciliary activity is observed. Subculture the fluid from the inoculated organ cultures into monolayer cultures to verify the isolation of virus, especially when the isolation in organ culture is in doubt.
9. Use of organ culture is likely to increase the number of rhinovirus isolates.

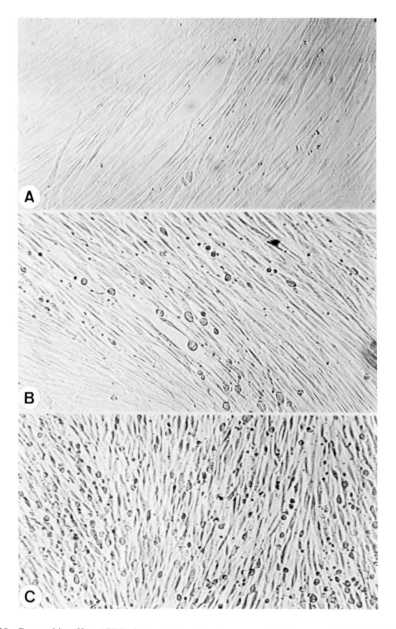

Figure 28. Cytopathic effect (CPE) induced by rhinovirus type 14 in human diploid fibroblastic cell culture WI-38 (100X).
A. Uninoculated WI-38 cell culture.
B. Early CPE, 24 hours after infection.
C. Late CPE, 72 hours after infection.

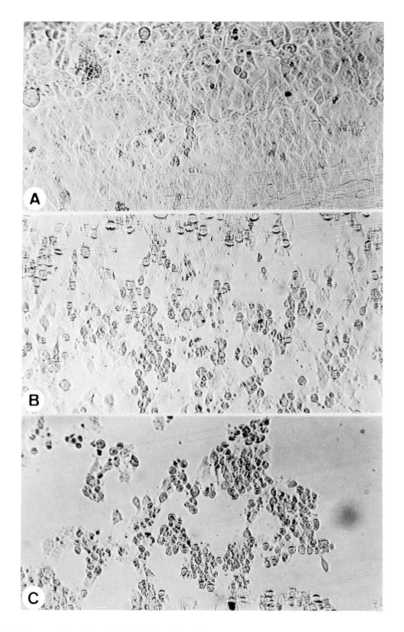

Figure 29. Cytopathic effect (CPE) induced by rhinovirus type 14 in HeLa cell culture (100X).
    A. Uninoculated HeLa cell culture.
    B. Early CPE, 24 hours after infection.
    C. Late CPE, 72 hours after infection.

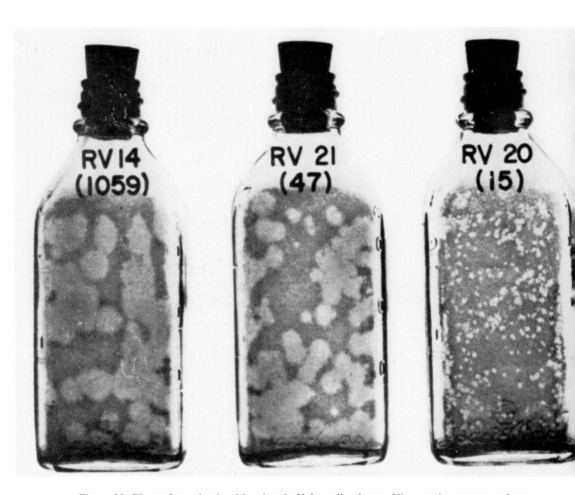

Figure 30. Plaque formation by rhinovirus in HeLa cell cultures. Virus strains represented are large, intermediate, and small plaque-formers (rhinoviruses 14, 21, and 20 respectively) (R. M. Conant et al., *Proc. Soc. Exp. Biol. Med.* 128: 51, 1968).

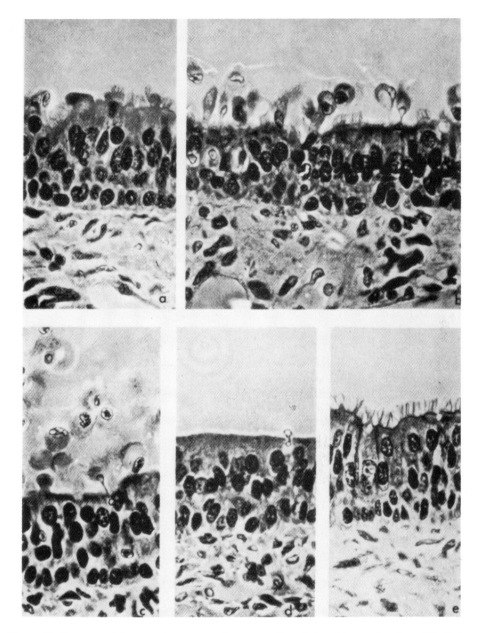

Figure 31. Progress of degenerative changes in organ culture induced by a rhinovirus, HS strain
(D. A. J. Tyrrell, *Virol. Mongr.* 2: 92, 1968).

    A. 18 hours after inoculation; most cells are well preserved, with a few single-ciliated
       cells.

    B. 24 hours after inoculation; many rounded cells are leaving the epithelial surface.

    C. 30 hours after inoculation; superficial cells appear disorganized.

    D. 58 hours after inoculation; most of the ciliated cells are gone.

    E. Uninfected culture fixed at the same time as D.

Identification of Isolates

pH stability test. The similarity of CPE induced by the rhinoviruses and by the enteroviruses sometimes necessitates determining that the isolate is not an enterovirus. Since the infectivity of a rhinovirus suspension treated at pH 3.0 is often reduced by 2 to 4 logs as compared to one without treatment, this characteristic provides a useful marker for separating the rhinoviruses from the enteroviruses. The latter are stable at low pH. In order to eliminate ether-sensitive viruses which are also acid pH sensitive, it is desirable to test for both ether-stability and acid-lability (see p. 82).

Neutralization test in tissue culture. Both CPE and plaque methods can be used to identify the rhinoviruses, by means of serum pools or type-specific antiserum. However, the growing number of serotypes greatly increases the labor necessary to perform a serologic identification.

Serodiagnosis

The situation is similar to that described for enteroviruses. Without virus isolation, serologic diagnosis is not practical. The neutralization test in tissue culture is the only method of testing acute and convalescent sera for antibody rises.

SUPPLEMENTARY READING

Enteroviruses

Books and Review Papers

Girst, N. R., Bell, E. J., and Assaad, F. Enteroviruses in human disease. *Prog. Med. Virol.* 24: 114, 1978.

Melnick, J. L., Wenner, H. A., and Phillips, C. A. Enteroviruses. In *Diagnostic procedures for viral, rickettsial and chlamydial infection,* ed. E. H. Lennette and N. J. Schmidt, p. 471. 5th ed. Washington, D. C.: American Public Health Association, 1979.

Specific Articles

Enders, J. F., Weller, T. H., and Robbins, F. C. Cultivation of the Lansing strain of poliomyelitis virus in cultures of various human embryonic tissues. *Science* 109: 85, 1949.

Herrmann, E. C., Jr., Person, D. A., and Smith, T. F. Experience in laboratory diagnosis of enterovirus infections in routine medical practice. *Mayo Clin. Proc.* 47: 577, 1972.

Hsiung, G. D. Application of primary cell culture in the study of animal viruses. III. Biological and genetic study of enteric viruses of man (enteroviruses). *Yale J. Biol. Med.* 33: 359, 1961.

Hsiung, G. D. Further studies on characterization and grouping of ECHO viruses—comparative virology. *Ann. N.Y. Acad. Sci.* 101: 413, 1962.

Landry, M. L., Madore, P., Fong, C. K. Y., and Hsiung, G. D. Use of guinea pig embryo cell cultures for isolation and propagation of group A coxsackieviruses. *J. Clin. Micro.* 13: 588, 1981.

Lim, K. A., and Benyesh-Melnick, M. Typing of viruses by combination of antiserum pools. Application to typing of enteroviruses (coxsackie and echo). *J. Immunol.* 84: 809, 1960.

Melnick, J. L., and Hampil, B. WHO collaborative studies on enterovirus reference antisera: fourth report. *Bull. W.H.O.* 48: 381, 1973.

Schmidt, N. J., Guenther, R. W., and Lennette, E. H. Typing of ECHO virus isolates by immune serum pools. The "intersecting serum scheme." *J. Immunol.* 87: 623, 1961.

Taber, L. H., Mirkovic, R. R., Adam, V., Ellis, S. S., Yow, M. D., and Melnick, J. L. Rapid diagnosis of enterovirus meningitis by immunofluorescent staining of CSF leukocytes. *Intervirol.* 1: 127, 1973.

Rhinoviruses

Books and Review Papers

Gwaltney, J. M., Jr. Rhinoviruses. In *Viral infections of humans, epidemiology and control*, ed. A. S. Evans, p. 383. New York: Plenum, 1976.

Hamparian, V. V. Rhinoviruses. In *Diagnostic procedures for viral, rickettsial, and chlamydial infections*, ed. E. H. Lennette and N. J. Schmidt, p. 535. 5th ed. Washington, D. C.: American Public Health Association, 1979.

Stott, E. J., and Killington, R. A. Rhinoviruses. *Ann. Rev. Micro.* 26: 503, 1972.

Tyrrell, D. A. Rhinoviruses. Virology Monogr. 2: 68, 1968.

Specific Articles

Cooney, M. K., and Kenny, G. E. Demonstration of dual rhinovirus infection in humans by isolation of different serotypes in human heteroploid (HeLa) and human diploid fibroblast cell cultures. *J. Clin. Micro.* 5: 202, 1977.

Fox, J. P., Cooney, M. K., and Hall, C. E. The Seattle virus watch. V. Epidemiology observations of rhinovirus infections 1965–1969 in families with young children. *Am. J. Epidemiol.* 101: 122, 1975.

Kapikian, A. Z., Almeida, J. D., and Scott, E. Immune electron microscopy of rhinoviruses. *J. Virol.* 10: 142, 1972.

Kapikian, A. Z., et al. A collaborative report: rhinovirus—extension of the numbering system. *Virology* 43: 524, 1971.

Lewis, F. A., and Kennett, M. L. Comparison of rhinovirus-sensitive HeLa cells and human embryo fibroblasts for isolations of rhinovirus from patients with respiratory disease. *J. Clin. Micro.* 3: 528, 1976.

13. Togaviridae*

ALPHAVIRUSES AND FLAVIVIRUSES

The togaviruses are examples of arthropod-borne viruses, or arboviruses. Since arboviruses are a group of highly heterogeneous viruses, only the togaviridae will be treated in this chapter. Members of the genera alphavirus and flavivirus within the family togaviridae originally were classified antigenically within arbovirus serologic groups A and B. By definition, an arbovirus is a virus that can be biologically transmitted by an arthropod vector. After the vector feeds on an infected vertebrate and virus multiplication occurs in the vector (the extrinsic incubation period), that vector is capable of transmitting the infection, by bite, to another vertebrate. This definition excludes those viruses that can be transmitted by arthropods but do not multiply in the vector. To date there are 446 registered arbovirus types, most of which are known or suspected to be arthropod-borne (table 14), but conclusive evidence for virus replication in a vector is available for relatively few. At present, arboviruses are classified on a serologic basis; any two or more viruses shown to be related but not identical serologically are considered to form a group.

Togaviruses share several physicochemical properties: they are small to medium in size (40–70 nm in diameter), are ether-sensitive, and contain single-stranded RNA. Their structures consist of a small icosahedral nucleocapsid and a lipid-containing envelope (figures 32 and 33). Replication of togaviruses occurs in the cytoplasm of infected cells; maturation and envelopment take place by budding at the plasma membrane (figure 32) or through intracytoplasmic membranes, most commonly the endoplasmic reticulum (figure 33).

In addition to the arthropod vectors, the most productive source for recovering togaviruses has been blood collected from humans and other animals during an acute phase of infection. Serologic methods are used for confirming the

*This chapter is contributed by N. Karabatsos of the Centers for Disease Control, Department of Health and Human Services, Fort Collins, Colorado.

diagnosis of an observed illness when paired sera are available and will be described in detail here because of their unique characteristics.

Although inoculation of newborn mice remains the method of choice for isolation of most important arboviruses, cell culture methods are important adjuncts. Table 15 lists the types of cell cultures that may be used for replication of certain arboviruses and the cytopathic effects (CPE) and plaque reactions that occur in these systems. There appears, however, to be some variation in the infectivity spectrum of these viruses and in their abilities to produce CPE and/or plaques in primary cell cultures as well as in serially propagated cell lines. These variations are influenced, at least to some degree, by the particular virus strain and the type of avian or mammalian cells from which the cultures were derived.

Specimen Inoculation

Sera from patients with acute febrile illnesses can be used undiluted for virus isolation or at dilutions of 1:10 and 1:100 in Medium-199 containing 5% fetal bovine serum (FBS). It is important to inoculate unknown specimens into mice at two or preferably more dilutions (undiluted to 10^{-3}), because some arboviruses, if inoculated at high concentrations, may induce potent inhibitors which restrict or completely mask symptoms of infection. In addition, a high concentration of defective particles in the specimen may induce "autointerference," while the presence of antibody in tissue specimens may disguise symptoms of the virus or produce a "prozone effect" at low dilutions.

When togavirus infection is a suspected cause of death, virus can generally be recovered from brain tissues taken at autopsy. Processed specimens should be inoculated into newborn mice or susceptible primary and serially propagated cell cultures with a minimum of delay, since these viruses are extremely labile when temperatures and pH vary.

Virus Isolation, Propagation, and Assay

Mouse pathogenicity. Until recently, the newborn mouse was considered a universal host system for the isolation of arboviruses. Newborn mice, 1 to 4 days old, are inoculated by intracranial (IC) route (0.01–0.02 ml) or in combination with intraperitoneal (IP) route (0.03–0.05 ml) (see figure 4). Except for a few alphaviruses that have an extremely short incubation period, illness or hindlimb paralysis usually occurs 2 to 5 days after inoculation. Mice showing signs of illness should be sacrificed immediately, brain tissue harvested, and a 10% suspension made in a buffered diluent containing 0.75% bovine albumin at a pH between 7.2 and 8.0. These brain suspensions are passed by the IC route to other suckling mice to confirm the isolation and for virus identification by serologic means.

In areas where arboviruses are endemic, mosquitoes are often trapped and used for virus isolation. Pools of up to 100 mosquitoes are ground in 2 ml of

Table 14. Registered Arboviruses, as of December 1981

Nucleic Acid Type	Virus Family and Genus	Particle Size (nm)	Serologic Group(s)	Total Number of Members	Commonly Known Virus Members
RNA	Togaviridae Alphavirus	70	A	25	eastern equine encephalitis western equine encephalitis Venezuelan equine encephalitis Sindbis
	Flavivirus	40–50	B	62	dengue 1–4 Japanese encephalitis St. Louis encephalitis tick-borne encephalitis West Nile yellow fever Powassan
	Possible members		Ungrouped	2	
	Bunyaviridae Bunyavirus	90–100	Bunyamwera supergroup; 16 serogroups + 1 serologically unassigned virus	111	Bunyamwera California encephalitis LaCrosse Oropouche
	Nairovirus		6 serogroups	22	Crimean hemorrhagic fever-Congo Nairobi sheep disease
	Phlebovirus		Phlebotomus fever serogroup	30	Naples sandfly fever Sicilian sandfly fever Rift Valley fever
	Uukuvirus		Uukuneimi serogroup	5	Uukuneimi
	"Bunyavirus-like" (unassigned or possible members)		7 serogroups + 14 ungrouped viruses	30	Bhanja

	Size	Serogroup	Number	Representative viruses
Orbivirus	65–80	11 serogroups + 9 ungrouped viruses	49	Colorado tick fever, bluetongue, Kemerovo, African horse sickness
Arenaviridae, Arenavirus	100–130	Tacaribe	9	Lassa, Junin, Machupo
Rhabdoviridae, Vesiculovirus	180×75	vesicular stomatitis virus serogroup	7	vesicular stomatitis, Indiana; vesicular stomatitis, New Jersey
Lyssavirus	180×75	rabies-related serogroup	1[a]	Lagos Bat[a]
Unassigned or possible members		5 serogroups + 20 ungrouped viruses	31	Hart Park, Flanders
Coronaviridae, Possible member	75–160	ungrouped	1	
Paramyxoviridae, Paramyxovirus	150	ungrouped	1	
Picornaviridae unclassified, possible member	22–30	ungrouped	1	
DNA				
Herpesviridae, Possible member	120–150	ungrouped	1	
Poxviridae, Possible members	300–450×170–260	ungrouped	2	
Iridoviridae, Unassigned	125–300	ungrouped	1	
Unclassified		5 serogroups + 45 ungrouped viruses	55	
		Total	446	

[a] Only 1 rabies-related virus is registered.

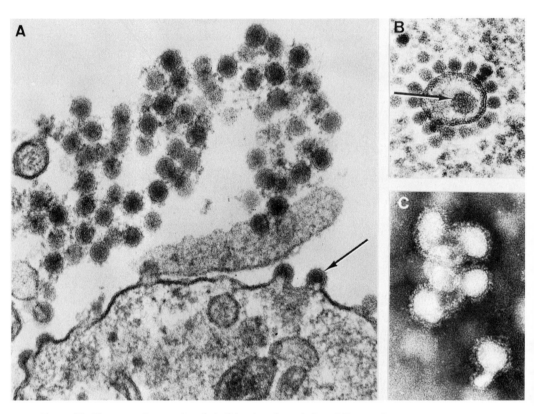

Figure 32. Electron micrographs of sindbis virus in an infected Vero cell.
      A. Thin section of sindbis virus–infected Vero cell showing extracellular virus parti-
      cles and nucleocapsids in the process of budding at the cell membrane (100,800X).
      B. Nucleocapsids and enveloped virus particle (arrow) in the cytoplasm of the cell
      (100,800X).
      C. Sindbis virus particles stained with PTA (168,000X).

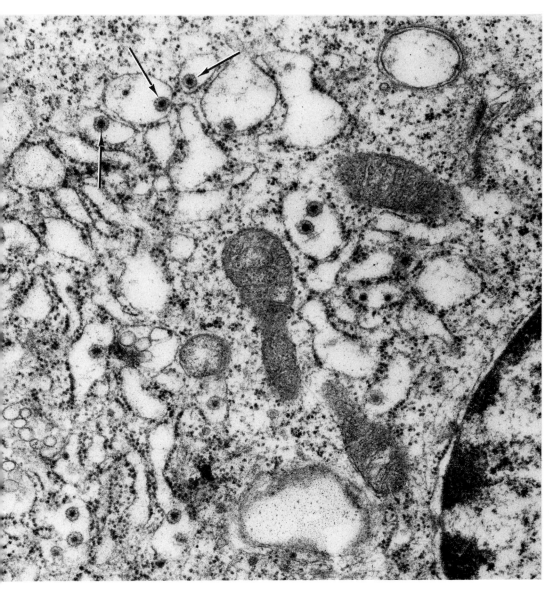

Figure 33. Electron micrograph of Japanese encephalitis virus in an infected BHK-21 cell, showing virus particles in the dilated endoplasmic reticulum (76,500X) (courtesy of J. D. Wright).

Table 15. Comparison of Cytopathic Effect[a] and Plaque Formation by Selected Arboviruses of Three Major Serogroups

Representative Virus Strains	Number of Days before Plaques Appear	Primary Cell Cultures						Passaged Cell Lines			
		Chick Embryo		Duck Kidney		Rhesus Monkey Kidney		BHK-21		Vero	
		CPE	Plaques	CPE	Plaques	CPE	Plaques	CPE	Plaques	CPE	Plaques
Alphavirus	2–3										
eastern equine encephalomyelitis		+	+	+	+	+	+	+	+	+	+
western equine encephalomyelitis		+	+	+	+	+	+	+	+	+	+
Venezuelan equine encephalomyelitis		+	+	+	+	+	+	+	+	+	+
Sindbis		+	+	+	+	−	+	+	+	+	+
Flavivirus	3–5										
St. Louis encephalitis		−	+	−	+	−	−	+	+	+	+
Japanese encephalitis		−	+	+	+	−	−	+	+[b]	+	+
West Nile		−	−	+	+	−	−	+	+	+	+
Bunyavirus	5–7										
Marituba		−	−	−	−	+/−	+	+	+	+	+
Oriboca		−	−	−	−	+/−	+	+	+	+	+
Apeu		−	−	−	−	+/−	+	+	+	+	+
Marutucu		−	−	−	−	+/−	+	+	+	+	+
Caraparu		−	−	−	−	+/−	+	+	+	+	+

[a]Appearance of cytopathic effect (CPE) may often be directly related to the concentration of virus inoculated.
[b]Test not done.

Key: + = virus-induced change
− = no change

116

Medium-199 containing 20% FBS and clarified by centrifugation at 12,100 × g for 30 minutes. Extracts of mosquitoes can be inoculated into mice or cell cultures as described above.

The sentinel mouse technique (exposure of newborn mice to mosquitoes in the field) has proven to be a useful procedure for isolating some arboviruses, especially in enzootic areas of the New World tropics. However, it is useful only in areas where virus-infected mosquitoes that feed on rodents are found. After exposure, the mice are observed in the laboratory for signs of illness, and sick mice are processed as above.

Cytopathic effect in cell cultures. Most of the togaviruses tested can be grown in both primary cell cultures and continuous cell lines. The primary cells most commonly used are chicken or duck embryo cell cultures, both of which are highly sensitive and readily available. Among the cell lines, Vero cells, an African green monkey kidney cell line, and BHK-21, a baby hamster kidney cell line, are frequently used. Insect cell cultures are increasingly being used with success. For example, mosquito cell cultures or intrathoracically-inoculated mosquitoes are even more sensitive for isolation of dengue viruses than is the rhesus monkey kidney cell line, LLC-MK$_2$. The latter, however, is preferred to newborn mice. In addition, mosquito cell cultures have been found to be more sensitive than newborn mice for isolation of yellow fever virus.

Cytopathic effect induced by eastern equine encephalomyelitis (EEE), Mayaro, and West Nile viruses in primary cell cultures is illustrated in figure 34. Unlike CPE caused by the enteroviruses, CPE induced by the togaviruses is generally not distinctive and cannot be used as a guide for presumptive diagnosis.

On the other hand, several flaviviruses have been reported to produce a distinctive CPE characterized by syncytium formation in continuous lines of mosquito cell cultures. These include Japanese encephalitis virus, West Nile virus and dengue virus types 1, 2, and 3. Other arboviruses that have been reported to produce CPE in invertebrate cell cultures include St. Louis encephalitis and yellow fever viruses, dengue virus type 4, an unidentified alphavirus, and an ungrouped flavivirus.

Plaque formation in cell cultures. Some togaviruses produce plaques but not CPE. Examples of plaques induced by a representative alphavirus (EEE), flavivirus (Ilheus), and bunyavirus (Oriboca) in Vero cells are shown in figure 35. In addition, certain alphaviruses also induce plaques in different primary cell cultures, incuding chicken embryo and duck kidney, but do so only poorly in primary rhesus monkey kidney (RhMK) cell monolayers (figure 36). Currently, plaque formation in flasks or plastic plates is used almost exclusively for virus assay and neutralization tests.

Hybridoma cell lines. An extremely important technological advancement took place relatively recently with the development of "hybridoma" cell lines, which secrete monospecific antibodies. Hybridoma cell lines are prepared by fusing splenic lymphocytes from immunized or hyperimmunized mice with mouse plasmacytoma cells. Clones of fused cells are isolated, and the antibodies

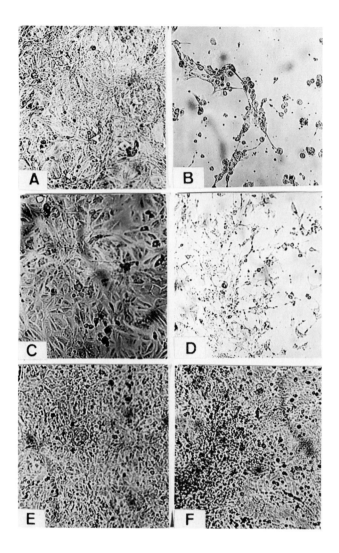

Figure 34. Cytopathic effect induced by representative togaviruses in primary cell cultures (100X) (J. R. Henderson, *Yale J. Biol. Med.* 33: 350, 1961).
  A. Uninoculated RhMK culture.
  B. Eastern equine encephalitis (EEE) virus–infected RhMK culture, 3 days after infection.
  C. Uninoculated guinea pig kidney culture.
  D. Mayaro virus–infected guinea pig kidney culture, 2 days after infection.
  E. Uninoculated duck embryo culture.
  F. West Nile virus–infected duck embryo culture, 5 days after infection.

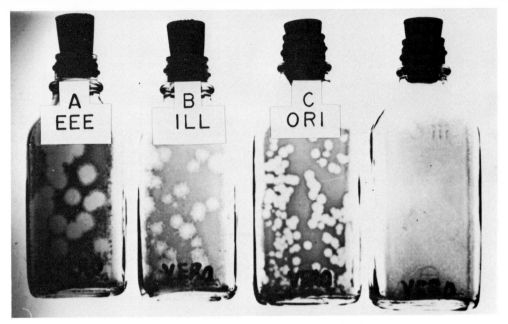

Figure 35. Plaque formation of representative togaviruses in Vero cell cultures.
    A. Eastern equine encephalitis virus.
    B. Ilheus virus.
    C. Oriboca virus.
    Bottle at right: Uninoculated control.

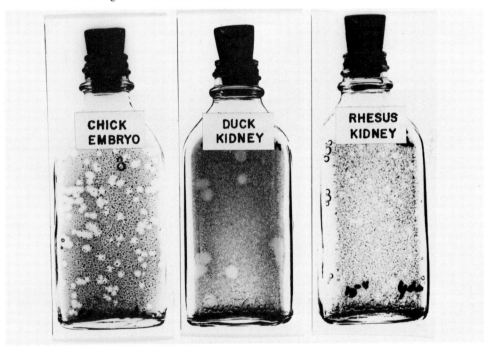

Figure 36. Plaque formation of Middleburg virus in primary cell cultures (J. R. Henderson, *Yale J. Biol. Med.* 33: 350, 1961). Left to right: Chicken embryo, 2 days after inoculation; duck kidney, 4 days after inoculation; rhesus monkey kidney, 4 days after inoculation.

secreted by these clones are characterized. Among the togaviruses, this important technology has been applied to analyzing and characterizing the antigenic structure of surface proteins of some of the important pathogens in this group. In addition, type-specific monoclonal dengue virus antibodies have been isolated and will be used to rapidly type and identify dengue isolates. Monoclonal antibodies also have been used to determine whether the antigenic domains involved in hemagglutination and in virus neutralization are different. Finally, they also have been used to define and analyze the antigenic relatedness among a cluster of viruses.

Identification of Isolates

The togaviruses are commonly identified by neutralization tests either in cell cultures (plaque-reduction neutralization) or in mice; hemagglutination-inhibition (HI), complement-fixation (CF), and immunofluorescent (IF) techniques have also been used since most alpha/flavi togaviruses possess common serogroup antigens as measured by one or more of the three tests. Cross-reactions are more evident in HI and less so in CF tests; most cross-reactions, but not all, are minimized by the neutralization test.

Mouse protection neutralization test. Neutralization tests in mice are often used for identification of togaviruses, particularly when an isolate is not known to propagate in a cell culture system. The procedures are similar to those described below for the plaque-reduction neutralization test.

Plaque-reduction neutralization test. Effective neutralization is often dependent upon a heat-labile factor; thus, fresh normal serum is added to the heat-inactivated test serum to enhance the neutralization test. Virus dilutions are made in phosphate-buffered saline (PBS) containing 0.75% bovine albumin; detailed procedures for plaque-reduction neutralization test are given in chapter 4.

Immunofluorescent staining reaction. The IF test is currently used as a rapid and accurate method for the identification of dengue viruses. The impression made from virus-infected salivary glands of mosquitoes is stained with fluorescein-conjugated dengue-immune serum. The direct IF test is described in chapter 9.

Hemagglutination-inhibition tests. Since hemagglutination activity by togaviruses is pH-dependent, the optimal pH must be determined each time the test is performed.

Preparation of HA Antigens from Infected Mouse Brain Tissue

1. Weigh infected mouse brain tissue and homogenize for 1 minute in a chilled electric blender (Sorvall Omni-mixer*) with 4 volumes of cold 8.5% sucrose in distilled water.
2. To 20 volumes of chilled acetone add 1 volume of homogenate by rap-

*Use of trade names is for identification only and does not constitute endorsement by the Public Health Service or by the U.S. Department of Health and Human Services.

idly dropping from a chilled syringe with large needle below the surface of the acetone.

3. Shake the mixture vigorously and allow tissue to settle for 10–30 minutes in a refrigerator.
4. Aspirate the supernatant and discard; add chilled acetone to the pink precipitate. The quantity of acetone added should be equal to the original volume of acetone used.
5. Shake vigorously and allow residue to settle for 60 minutes at 4°C.
6. Remove and discard the supernatant fluid; add a small quantity of fresh acetone to the sediment to remove extracted tissue.
7. Transfer sediment to thick-walled centrifuge bottles immersed in an ice bath and dry by attaching to a vacuum pump for 2.5 hours.
8. Rehydrate the dried sediment with borate saline, pH 9.0, in a volume equal to 0.4 of the volume of the original homogenate; let stand overnight in the refrigerator.
9. Centrifuge the rehydrated preparation at 12,100 $\times$ g for 30 minutes.

The supernatant fluid representing the finished hemagglutinating antigen can be stored in the frozen state or lyophilized. Since sucrose exerts a protective effect, all sucrose-acetone-extracted antigens contain residual infective virus. If serology is to be performed with an inactivated antigen, proceed from step 7 above as follows:

8. Rehydrate the dried sediment with borate saline, pH 9.0, containing 0.1M Tris buffer in a volume equal to 0.4 of the volume of the original homogenate; let stand overnight in refrigerator.
9. Centrifuge the rehydrated preparation at 12,100 $\times$ g for 30 minutes.
10. Prepare a 10% solution of beta-propiolactone (BPL) in cold PBS. Add sufficient BPL to antigen to give a final concentration of 0.3% for the inactivation of alphaviruses. A final concentration of 0.1% BPL is used to treat flavivirus antigen preparations. Stir antigen mixture for 72 hours at 4°C.
11. Test for loss of infectivity by inoculation of newborn mice.

Titration of the HA Antigen at Different pH Values

1. Prepare serial two-fold dilutions of HA antigen in borate-buffered saline, pH 9.0, containing 0.4% bovine serum albumin (formula below). Each dilution should be represented by a volume of 0.05 ml.
2. To test for HA activity at several different pH values, prepare several identical sets of antigen dilutions in plastic panels, using pH-adjusting diluents (formula below).
3. Prepare a working suspension of goose red blood cells (RBC) by diluting the 8% stock suspension (prepared in dextrose gelatin veronal (DGV) diluent; formula below) to 1:24 in the various pH-adjusting diluents (pH 5.8 to 7.0 in increments of 0.1 pH unit).
4. Add 0.05 ml of the working RBC suspension to each of the antigen dilu-

tions in the plastic panels and cover with a plastic sheet. Also include a set of RBC in diluents of different pH values as controls. Incubate at 22°C or at room temperature for 60 minutes or until RBC settle.

5. The highest antigen dilution showing complete agglutination is taken as the end point. The optimal pH is that yielding the highest HA titer and clearest HA pattern.
6. Calculate the dilution at the optimal pH that gives 8–16 units per 0.05 ml or 4–8 units per 0.025 ml.

Hemgglutination-inhibition test. Determine the pH at which the antigen is optimally reactive and the approximate titer of the preparation. The antigen is then tested against antisera to recognized viruses. It is essential to include homologous titrations with known antigen and the same known antisera for comparison.

1. Prepare serial two-fold dilutions of serum, which has been pretreated with kaolin or acetone to remove inhibitors, in borate-buffered saline containing 0.4% bovine albumin, pH 9.0.
2. Dilute the HA antigen to contain 8 units per 0.025 ml. The dilution necessary to give this number of units is calculated from the titer at that pH showing the highest HA activity.
3. Add 0.025 ml of the virus antigen containing 8 HA units to 0.025 ml of each dilution of serum; incubate at room temperature for 2 hours, keeping the plate covered during this period.
4. Dilute an 8% suspension of male domestic goose erythrocytes to 1:24 in the adjusting diluent that yields the optimal pH for HA activity. Add 0.05 ml of the diluted RBC suspension to each virus-antibody mixture.
5. Prepare 3 controls: serum with diluent and RBC (serum control); diluent plus RBC (cell control); and a titration of the diluted HA preparation for verifying the exact number of units employed (antigen control).
6. Incubate test and homologous titrations, as well as the serum controls, cell controls, and antigen controls, at room temperature for 30–60 minutes. The end-point titers are read as the highest dilutions of serum completely inhibiting the agglutination of 8 HA units of antigen.

Removal of Nonspecific Inhibitors in Sera by Acetone Treatment

1. Dilute sera to 1:10 with PBS.
2. Chill diluted serum in an ice bath and add 12 volumes of cold acetone.
3. Extract for 5 minutes with periodic shaking.
4. Centrifuge for 5 minutes at 11,060 × g and remove the supernatant by aspiration.
5. Reextract the precipitate as before.
6. Aspirate the acetone and dry the sediment for 2 hours with a vacuum pump or allow to air-dry overnight at room temperature.
7. Reconstitute the dried material in borate saline, pH 9.0, to give the equivalent of a 1:10 serum dilution.

8. To remove naturally occurring agglutinins for goose erythrocytes, chill treated sera in an ice bath and add 0.1 ml of packed, washed goose RBC per 5 ml of serum at the 1:10 dilution.
9. Allow adsorption to take place for 20 minutes with occasional shaking.
10. Centrifuge for 10 minutes at 400 × g in the cold. Remove supernatant fluid and test the HI reaction.

Serodiagnosis

The HI, neutralization, and CF tests are used for presumptive diagnosis of togavirus infection in recently ill patients from whom no virus was isolated during the acute phase. The CF antibody titer rises more slowly than the HI and the neutralizing antibodies, but decreases rapidly, usually within a few months. Thus, the HI and neutralization tests can be used for detection of IgM or IgG, whereas the CF test can only detect IgG antibody.

There are several other tests which are used for the measurement of arboviral antibodies. Some of these tests were developed relatively recently and, in general, have been shown to be more sensitive and rapid than some of the older, conventional serologic procedures. In some instances their usefulness is limited by the expense associated with the use of radioactive substances and by the necessity to use purified viral reagents. The enzyme-linked immunosorbent assay (ELISA) is a highly sensitive, objective, and rapid test which does not require the use of radioactive substances. The test, which usually requires the use of purified or partially purified viral antigens, is basically a combining assay and, therefore, requires only the combination of antibody with antigen. It can be used to measure antibody in either the IgG or IgM classes. The radioimmunoassay (RIA) is also a rapid, objective, and sensitive test which can be applied to the measurement of antibody in the different immunoglobulin classes. This test also measures antigen-antibody combination on a solid phase. It usually requires the use of purified or partially purified viral antigenic components, and radioactive substances, with a limited shelf-life, are routinely employed in this test procedure. The immunofluorescence assay (IFA) is a simple, inexpensive test which has been shown to be as specific as and more sensitive than the HI test for the serologic diagnosis of certain flavivirus infections. Furthermore, this test procedure has been recommended as the procedure of choice for the serologic diagnosis of Lassa fever virus infections. Although it was found to be less time-consuming and more sensitive than the CF test, it is somewhat subjective, labor-intensive, and does not readily lend itself to automation.

Acute and convalescent sera are used for antibody determinations. A fourfold or greater rise or fall in antibody titer to a given virus is presumptive evidence that the virus used in the test or a related virus was responsible for the illness. Since infection with some arboviruses induces antibody responses that persist for many years, perhaps for life, antibody determinations in a given population can be used for determining prevalence of infections.

REAGENTS

Borate-Buffered Saline, pH 9.0

The final solution consists of 0.05M borate–0.12M NaCl. Prepare by diluting with distilled water 80 ml 1.5M NaCl, 100 ml of 0.05M H_3BO_3, and 23 ml 1.0M NaOH to 1 liter.

pH-Adjusting Diluents for Arbovirus HA Test

The following tabulation gives the percentage combinations of phosphate buffers. Each combination (A + B) when mixed with an equal volume of borate saline, pH 9.0 (above), gives the final pH indicated in the tabulation.

Solution A (in ml) 0.15M NaCl– 0.2M Na_2HPO_4	Solution B (in ml) 0.15M NaCl– 0.2M NaH_2PO_4	Final pH
3.0	97.0	5.75
12.5	87.5	6.0
22.0	78.0	6.2
32.0	68.0	6.4
45.0	55.0	6.6
55.0	45.0	6.8
64.0	36.0	7.0
72.0	28.0	7.2
79.0	21.0	7.4

Dextrose Gelatin Veronal (DGV)

Veronal (barbital)	0.58 gm
Gelatin	0.60 gm
Sodium veronal (sodium barbital)	0.38 gm
$CaCl_2$ (anhydrous)	0.02 gm
$MgSO_4 \cdot 7H_2O$	0.12 gm
NaCl	8.5 gm
Dextrose	10.0 gm
Distilled water	1000.0 ml

The veronal and gelatin are dissolved in water by heating. Other reagents are added and the mixture is autoclaved at 10 lbs. for 10 minutes.

SUPPLEMENTARY READING

Books and Review Papers

Berge, T. O., ed. *International catalogue of arboviruses*. 2nd ed. DHEW publication No. (CDC) 75–8301. Washington, D.C.: U.S. Government Printing Office, 1975.
Monath, T. P., ed. *St. Louis encephalitis*. Washington, D.C.: American Public Health Association, 1980.

Mussgay, M., Enzman, P. J., Horzinek, M. C., and Weiland, E. Growth cycle of arboviruses in vertebrate and arthropod cells. *Progr. Med. Virol.* 19: 257, 1975.

Schlesinger, R. W., ed. *The togaviruses: biology, structure, replication.* New York: Academic Press, 1980.

Theiler, M., and Downs, W. G. *The arthropod-borne viruses of vertebrates: an account of the Rockefeller Foundation virus program, 1951–1970.* New Haven: Yale University Press, 1973.

Specific Articles

American Committee on Arthropod-Borne Viruses. Arbovirus names. *Am. J. Trop. Med. Hyg.* 18: 731, 1969.

Bishop, D. H. L., et al. Bunyaviridae. *Intervirology* 14: 125, 1980.

Brand, O. M., and Allen, W. P. Preparation of noninfectious arbovirus antigens. *Appl. Microbiol.* 20: 298, 1970.

Dittmar, D., Haines, H. G., and Castro, A. Monoclonal antibodies specific for dengue virus type 3. *J. Clin. Microbiol.* 12: 74, 1980.

French, G. R., and McKinney, R. W. Use of Beta-propiolactone in preparation of inactivated arbovirus serologic test antigens. *J. Immunol.* 92: 772, 1964.

Gentry, M. K., Henchal, E. A., McCown, J. M., Brandt, W. E., and Dalrymple, J. M. Identification of distinct antigenic determinants on dengue-2 virus using monoclonal antibodies. *Am. J. Trop. Med. Hyg.* 31: 548, 1982.

Hofmann, H., Frisch-Niggemeyer, W., and Heinz, F. Rapid diagnosis of tick-borne encephalitis by means of enzyme-linked immunosorbent assay. *J. Gen. Virol.* 42: 505, 1979.

Karabatsos, N. Supplement to the international catalogue of arboviruses. *Am. J. Trop. Med. Hyg.* 27: 372, 1978.

Klimas, R. A., Ushijima, H., Clerx-Van Haaster, C. M., and Bishop, D. H. L. Radioimmune assays and molecular studies that place anopheles B and Turlock serogroup viruses in the Bunyavirus genus (Bunyaviridae). *Am. J. Trop. Med. Hyg.* 30: 876, 1981.

Matthews, R. E. F. Classification and nomenclature of viruses. *Intervirology* 12: 132, 1979.

Nagarkatti, P. S., and Nagarkatti, M. Comparison of hemagglutination-inhibition (HI) and indirect fluorescent antibody (IFA) techniques for the serological diagnosis of certain flavivirus infections. *J. Trop. Med. Hyg.* 83: 115, 1980.

Peiris, J. S. M., Porterfield, J. S., and Roehrig, J. T. Monoclonal antibodies against the flavivirus West Nile. *J. Gen. Virol.* 58: 283, 1982.

Roehrig, J. T., Corser, J. A., and Schlesinger, M. J. Isolation and characterization of hybrid cell lines producing monoclonal antibodies directed against the structural proteins of Sindbis virus. *Virology* 101: 41, 1980.

Roehrig, J. T., Gorski, D., and Schlesinger, M. J. Properties of monoclonal antibodies directed against the glycoproteins of Sindbis virus. *J. Gen. Virol.* In press.

Rosen, L., and Gubler, D. J. The use of mosquitoes to detect and propagate dengue viruses. *Am. J. Trop. Med. Hyg.* 23: 1153, 1974.

Subcommittee on Arbovirus Laboratory Safety of the American Committee on Arthropod-Borne Viruses. Laboratory safety for arboviruses and certain other viruses of vertebrates. *Am. J. Trop. Med. Hyg.* 29: 1359, 1980.

Trent, D. W., Harvey, C. L., Qureshi, A., and LeStourgeon, D. Solid-phase radioimmunoassay for antibodies to flavivirus structural and nonstructural proteins. *Infect. and Immun.* 13: 1325, 1976.

Varma, M. G. R., Pudney, M., Leake, C. J., and Peralta, P. H. Isolation in a mosquito (*Aedes pseudoscutellaris*) cell line (Mos. 61) of yellow fever virus strains from original field material. *Intervirology* 6: 50, 1975/6.

Wulff, H., and Lange, J. V. Indirect immunofluorescence for the diagnosis of Lassa fever infection. *Bull. W.H.O.* 52: 429, 1975.

14. Rubiviridae

RUBELLA VIRUS

Rubella virus is the etiological agent of German measles, a common and benign disease of children. Clinically, the patient starts with mild upper-respiratory symptoms followed by enlarged lymph nodes of the neck and finally a generalized rash which lasts 2 to 3 days. This disease, however, is of great significance when it occurs in pregnant women, especially during the first trimester, since it frequently gives rise to congenital defects in the infant.

The rubella virion is spherical and approximately 60 nm in diameter (figure 37). Negative staining preparations reveal an envelope but the nucleocapsid symmetry is obscure. Multiplication of rubella virus is not inhibited by 5-bromo-2′-deoxyuridine, indicating its nucleic acid constituent is RNA. Like other viruses with lipid envelopes, rubella virus is rapidly inactivated by ether, chloroform, or sodium deoxycholate. The virus is relatively labile but can be stored at $-70°C$ for prolonged periods.

Rubella virus replicates in a variety of primary cell cultures and passaged diploid cell strains but, in general, cellular degeneration is not readily observed in the infected cultures. The manifestation of CPE appears to depend upon the cell culture type, the serum concentration in the medium, and the amount of vitamins and/or amino acids present. In infected primary green MK cell cultures, evidence of virus growth can be determined by an interference phenomenon, that is, interference with the growth of a challenge virus. Cytopathic effect, however, has been observed in several other cell systems infected with rubella virus. These include a baby hamster kidney cell line (BHK-21), rabbit kidney cell line (RK-13), and an African green monkey kidney cell line (Vero cells). After two or three passages in BHK-21 cell cultures, a hemagglutinin titer can be detected in the infected culture fluid. It should be noted that the ability of cell lines to demonstrate rubella virus–induced CPE varies greatly from cell line to cell line and from laboratory to laboratory. Maintenance of

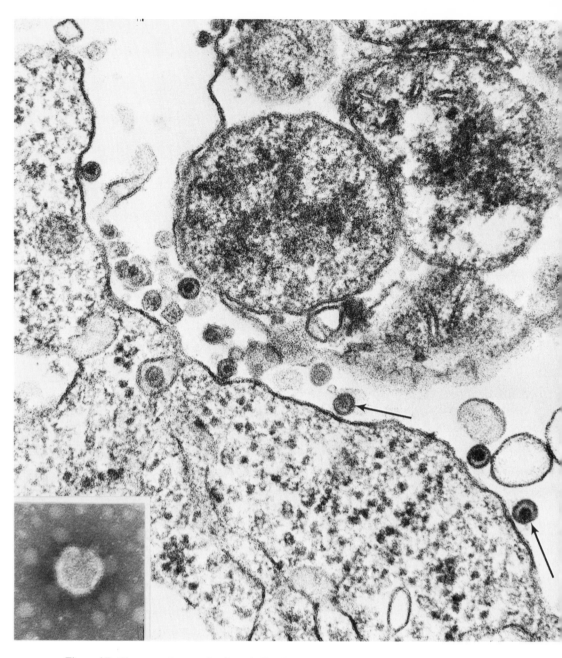

Figure 37. Electron micrograph of a rubella virus–infected Vero cell, showing mature virus particles at the extracellular space (100,800X). Inset: Virus particles stained with PTA (168,000X).

inoculated BHK-21 cells until CPE induced by the slow-growing rubella virus is often difficult; however, inoculation of the BHK-21 cells while in suspension and testing by IP staining 4–5 days after seeding of the infected cells appears to be satisfactory.

Specimen Inoculation

Throat swabs or washings, acute phase blood, cerebrospinal fluid, urine, amniotic fluid, and placental and fetal tissues are all useful for isolation of rubella virus. Primary African green monkey kidney cell cultures, human amnion, RK-13, and BHK-21 cells are commonly used for inoculation of specimens, although other cell lines including Vero or BSC-1 green monkey kidney cell line also can be used.

Virus Isolation, Propagation, and Assay

Interference in African green monkey kidney cell cultures. Primary GMK cultures infected with rubella virus show no evidence of CPE. However, a rubella virus–infected culture will not support the growth of added echovirus type 11. This interference phenomenon was one of the methods originally used for the detection of rubella virus, as the inhibition of echovirus type 11–induced CPE indicates the presence of an interfering agent. Other virus types, including poliovirus type 1, coxsackie virus A-9, vesicular stomatitis virus (VSV), and Newcastle disease virus (NDV), have also been used as challenge viruses. Despite the difficulties encountered with the interference method, which requires an additional step for detection, the interference phenomenon in primary GMK cultures is still the most reliable and sensitive procedure for detecting the presence of rubella virus.

Cytopathic effect in primary human amnion cell cultures. The first observation of rubella virus–induced CPE in human amnion cell cultures was made under certain strict conditions. The cultures were in excellent condition with uniform cell sheets; the medium consisted of 45% bovine amniotic fluid, 45% Hanks' BSS, 5% bovine embryo extract, and 5% horse serum; and the cultures were incubated at 35°C in a roller drum. Adherence to these conditions is necessary to maintain the cultures for the 30 days required for development of CPE, which begins with dissolution of isolated cells that gradually spreads to involve the entire cell sheet (figure 38A–E). Staining with hematoxylin and eosin reveals eosinophilic inclusions (figure 38F). Interference can also be demonstrated in rubella virus–infected human amnion cells challenged with Sindbis virus.

Cytopathic effect in rabbit kidney cells. Primary rabbit kidney cells or passaged cell lines have been used for isolation of rubella virus; CPE has been observed in RK-13 cell cultures (figure 39). The microplaques produced are more easily seen under a phase-contrast microscope. Appearance of distinct

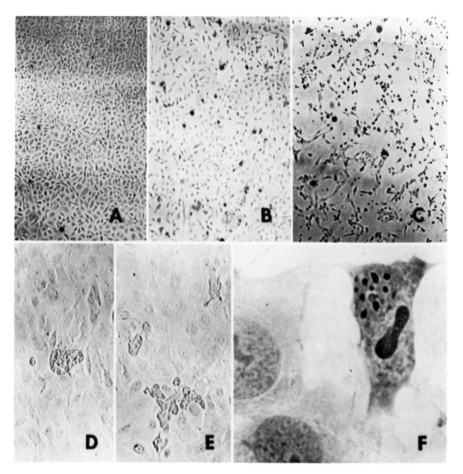

Figure 38. Cytopathic effect induced by rubella virus in human amnion cell cultures (A, B, C, wet preparations, 100X; D, E, F, stained preparations, 400X) (F. A. Neva et al., *Bact. Rev.* 28: 446, 1964).
  A. Uninfected normal human amnion cell culture.
  B. Rubella virus–infected culture, 14 days after inoculation.
  C. Rubella virus–infected culture, 24 days after inoculation.
  D. Single infected cell with adjacent uninvolved cells, 10 days after inoculation.
  E. Scattered infected cells showing ameboid distortion, 10 days after inoculation.
  F. Infected cell with large eosinophilic cytoplasmic inclusions and basophilic aggregation of nuclear chromatin as well as portions of two normal cells.

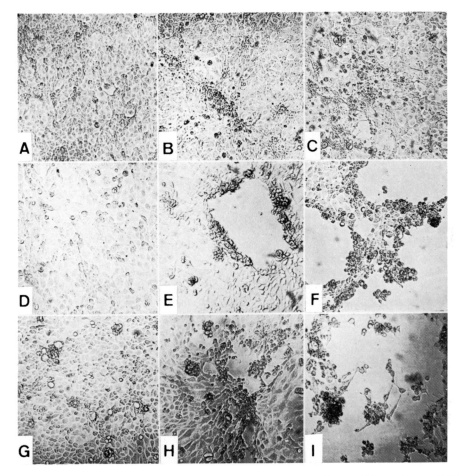

Figue 39. Cytopathic effect induced by rubella virus in rabbit kidney cell line cultures (100X)
(J. Furesz et al., *Canad. J. Microbiol.* 15: 71, 1969).
A–C. RK-13 microcultures. (A) Uninoculated cultures; (B) 5 days; (C) 8 days after
inoculation with HP-78 rubella virus.
D–F. RK1-H microcultures. (D) Uninoculated cultures; (E) 5 days; (F) 8 days after
inoculation of the same virus.
G–I. RK1-FC microcultures. (G) Uninoculated cultures; (H) 5 days; (I) 8 days after
inoculation of the same virus.

CPE often requires 7 days or more of cultivation and, occasionally, 2 or 3 serial blind passages of culture fluid may be necessary.

Plaque formation in passaged cell lines. Rubella virus induces clear sharp plaques in Vero cells and RK-13 cell cultures. Plaques appear 7 to 8 days after infection; they are round with ragged edges and measure 2 to 3 mm in diameter, increasing in size after prolonged incubation. This method is not used for primary virus isolation but is used frequently for virus assay and antibody detection.

Isolation of virus from fetal tissues. Isolation of rubella virus from fetal specimens is most successfully accomplished by cultivation or cocultivation of intact infected cells. The fetal tissues are trypsinized (for procedure, see p. 249) to obtain a cell suspension and the intact cells either are seeded in growth medium for propagation into cell sheets or are cocultivated with susceptible cell monolayers; the cultured cells and fluids thus obtained provide good sources for virus stocks.

Identification of Isolates

If clinical material is being examined specifically for rubella virus and the isolate is made in RK-13 cells, confirmation should be made by subculture of the infected material into primary GMK cell cultures and challenged with echovirus type 11 or other virus. If a suspected rubella virus is isolated in a Vero cell culture, one can perform the interference neutralization test in the same cell line, although subculture into primary GMK culture is preferable.

Neutralization test in tissue culture. This test is the most specific for identification of a suspected rubella virus isolate.

1. The isolate is diluted in serial 10-fold dilutions up to 10^{-6} and each dilution is inoculated into three tubes, 0.1 ml per tube, for the determination of infectivity titers.
2. Add an equal volume of a constant amount of known rubella antiserum to each dilution of virus, and allow the mixture to stand at 37°C for 1 hour.
3. Inoculate 0.2 ml of each mixture into a culture tube, 3 to 4 tubes per dilution.
4. If the cell system is one in which the rubella causes CPE, e.g. RK-13, the inoculated cultures are read at intervals until cultures that do not contain rubella antiserum show CPE.
5. If an interference-producing cell system is used, e.g. the GMK cell cultures, the challenge virus is added routinely at 7 days. A 100 to 1000 $TCID_{50}$ of echovirus type 11 is commonly used as a challenge dose and is added to each culture tube, with or without rubella antiserum. A positive neutralization test is indicted when those tubes inoculated with virus-serum mixture show *no* interference, that is, when CPE of echovirus type 11 is evident.

Hemagglutination-inhibition test. In the preparation of rubella HA antigen, it is necessary to remove inhibitors from the serum that is used in the maintenance medium for rubella virus–infected cell cultures. The maintenance medium for BHK-21 cell cultures consists of 2% fetal bovine serum which can be treated with kaolin to remove nonspecific inhibitors in the serum. Therefore rubella HA antigen obtained from serum containing BHK-21 cell culture fluid can be extracted directly with Tween 80 and ether treatment. Antigen from rubella-infected BHK-21 cultures maintained with 0.4% bovine albumin can be used without further treatment. Rubella HA antigen is stable indefinitely when stored at $-60°C$. Procedures for the HA and HI tests are described in chapter 5; but to test for the presence of rubella virus hemagglutinin, 0.5% day-old chick, adult goose, or pigeon RBC in PBS are used, and the reaction takes place at 4°C or 22°C but not at 37°C. Calcium is essential for the agglutination of RBC by rubella virus. Inhibition of chick RBC agglutination by the virus in the presence of immune serum identifies rubella virus.

Immunofluorescent or immunoperoxidase staining method. These methods provide more rapid alternatives to the neutralization test.

1. Subculture rubella virus isolates into Leighton tubes containing cover-slips, with the same cell type in which they were isolated.
2. Five to seven days after inoculation, remove culture fluids and air-dry the infected cells on coverslips at room temperature.
3. Fix the infected cells on coverslips with cold acetone and keep at $-20°C$ for 30 minutes; air-dry at room temperature. (These fixed cells can be stored at $-60°C$ until used.)
4. Prior to the test, known immune and preimmune rabbit sera are inactivated at 56°C for 30 minutes and adsorbed with 20% normal mouse brain to reduce nonspecific staining.
5. For the identification of rubella virus the indirect IP or IF methods in chapters 8 and 9 can be used. The fluorescent or enzyme-conjugated anti-rabbit globulin prepared in goat can be obtained commercially.

Electron microscopy. Electron microscopic examination of rubella virus–infected cells reveals that virus replication occurs in the cytoplasm and that virus particle envelopment takes place by budding at the plasma membrane or into cytoplasmic vacuoles (figure 37). Examination of negatively stained virus particles by electron microscope is not a routine procedure since the structure of the rubella virus particle in a nonpurified preparation is not easily distinguishable from cellular material.

Serodiagnosis

Since the procedures used for rubella virus isolation can be time-consuming and tedious, serologic tests are commonly applied for establishing evidence of recent rubella virus infection. Several methods have been established for detecting rubella virus antibody, including HI, CF, neutralization, immunoperoxidase, and

Table 16. Suggested Tests for Rubella Virus Antibodies

| Clinical Situation | Choice of Serologic Test | | Interpretation |
	1st	2nd	
Paired serum samples from patient with rash First serum taken within one week of onset Convalescent serum taken 14–21 days after onset	HI	CF	A 4-fold rise confirms recent infection.
Single serum samples taken following acute illness	HI-IgM	CF	Presence of antibody in the IgM fraction suggests recent infection.
Exposure/no illness: Serum taken within 7 days (follow-up serum if negative, especially for pregnant women)	HI	CF	Presence of HI antibody titers≥10 indicates past infection and thus immunity to primary rubella.
Suspicion of congenital rubella: Infants<3 months of age (follow-up serum needed)	HI-IgM	NT	Presence of antibody in the IgM fraction suggests congenital infection.
Infants 3–6 months of age (infant and maternal sera needed)	HI	NT	Presence of antibody suggests congenital infection if infant's titer is significantly higher than mother's titer.
Infants 6–12 months of age	HI	NT	Presence of antibody suggests congenital infection if infant has not been exposed to rubella virus.

immunofluorescence. The clinical importance of a serodiagnosis of rubella virus infection has stimulated commercial suppliers to prepare almost all the reagents needed for the various serologic tests. Table 16 presents alternative methods for rubella antibody testing under different clinical circumstances.

Hemagglutination-inhibition test is the method most widely used in the laboratory for diagnosis of rubella virus infection. Although the HI test described in chapter 5 can be applied, the impact of variables on HI test results are often encountered. Thus the type of RBC, the concentration of antigen, the composition of the diluent, the method used for removing nonspecific inhibitors, and the temperature of incubation can all affect the outcome. The following procedures describe the variables that have been identified as critical when adapting the HI test to rubella virus serodiagnosis.

1. *Treatment of serum.* Serum samples may be inactivated at 56°C for 30 minutes, although noninactivated serum can be used. Serum must be treated with kaolin, preferably with heparin-$MnCl_2$ (for formula, see below), to remove the nonspecific B-lipoprotein inhibitors; adsorption with chick RBC to remove natural cell agglutinin is also recommended.
2. *Choice of erythrocytes.* Although RBC from a variety of species can be used, 1- to 3-day-old chick RBC are preferred for testing rubella virus hemagglutinin.
3. *Composition of diluent.* HSAG diluent, or Hepes (N-2-hydroxyethyl-piperazine-N' ethane sulphonic acid)-saline-albumin-gelatin, at pH 6.2 is used for rubella HA test (formula below). The reaction is enhanced by the presence of 0.001M $CaCl_2$.

Determination of IgM antibody. Demonstration of specific IgM antibody to rubella virus is a valuable aid in serologic diagnosis of rubella infection. Several techniques are available to separate IgM. These include absorption with staphylococcal protein A to remove IgG or sucrose gradient centrifugation to separate IgM from IgG. Additional techniques using IgM antiglobulin are available in the indirect IF or ELISA test.

REAGENTS

MnCl₂ 1M Solution

$MnCl_2 \cdot 4H_2O$	39.6 gm
Distilled water, demineralized	200.0 ml

Sterilize by millipore membrane filtration and store in the dark at 4°C. Discard if brown precipitate appears. To prepare a working solution of heparin-$MnCl_2$ solution, mix equal parts of heparin (5000 units per ml) and 1M $MnCl_2$. Store at 4°C and use in two weeks.

Hepes Saline 5X Stock Solution

Hepes	29.80 gm
NaCl	40.95 gm
$CaCl_2 \cdot 2H_2O$	0.74 gm
Distilled water, demineralized	1000 ml

Sterilize by filtration through millipore membrane and store at 4°C.

Bovine Serum Albumin 2X Stock Solution

Bovine albumin powder (Fraction V)   20.0 gm
Distilled water, demineralized   1000 ml
Sterilize by filtration through millipore membrane and store at 4°C.

Gelatin 10X Stock Solution

Gelatin   25.0 gm
Distilled water, demineralized   1000 ml
Dissolve the gelatin and sterilize the solution at 15 lbs. for 15 minutes; store at 4°C.

HSAG Diluent Working Solution

Hepes saline 5X stock solution   200 ml
Bovine serum albumin 2X stock solution   500 ml
Gelatin 10X stock solution   100 ml
Distilled water, demineralized   200 ml
Adjust the pH to 6.2. This solution can be stored at 4°C for 2 months.

SUPPLEMENTARY READING

Books and Review Papers

Palmer, D. F., Herrmann, K. L., Lincoln, R. E., Hearn, M. V., and Fuller, M. J., eds. *A procedural guide to the performance of the rubella hemagglutination-inhibition test.* Center for Disease Control and Immunity Series No. 2. Atlanta, Ga., 1970.

Parkman, P. D., Hopps, H. E., and Meyer, H. M., Jr. Rubiviridae (rubella virus). In *Virology and rickettsiology* ed. G. D. Hsiung and R. H. Green, vol. 1, pt. 1, p. 201. Handbook series in clinical laboratory science, Section H. West Palm Beach, Fla.: CRC Press, 1978.

Specific Articles

Ankerst, I., Christensen, P., Kjellen, L., and Kronvall, G. A routine diagnostic test for IgA and IgM antibodies to rubella virus: adsorption of IgG with staphylococcus aureus. *J. Infect. Dis.* 130: 268, 1974.

Gravell, M., Procett, P. H., Gutenson, O., and Ley, A. C. Detection of antibody to rubella virus by enzyme-linked immunosorbent assay. *J. Infect. Dis.* 136: 5300, 1977.

Fenner, F. Classification and nomenclature of viruses, second report of the international committee on taxonomy of viruses. *Intervirology* 7: 44, 1976.

Parkman, P. D., Buescher, E. L., and Artenstein, M. S. Recovery of rubella virus from army recruits. *Proc. Soc. Biol. Med.* 111: 225, 1962.

Schmidt, N. J., Ho, H. H., and Chin, J. Application of immunoperoxidase staining to more rapid detection and identification of rubella virus isolates. *J. Clinical Micro.* 13: 627, 1981.

Van der Logt, J. T. M., Van Loon, A. M., and Van der Veen, J. Hemadsorption immunosorbent technique for determination of rubella immunoglobulin M antibody. *J. Clin. Micro.* 13: 410, 1981.

Voller, A., and Bidwell, D. E. A simple method for detecting antibodies to rubella. *Br. J. Exp. Path.* 56: 338, 1975.

Weller, T. H., and Neva, F. A. Propagation in tissue culture of cytopathic agents in patients with rubella-like illness. *Proc. Soc. Exp. Biol. Med.* 111: 215, 1962.

15. Myxoviridae

INFLUENZA AND PARAINFLUENZA VIRUSES

The myxovirus group includes influenza, parainfluenza, and mumps viruses of man and Newcastle disease virus of poultry (table 17). The latter three are now referred to as the paramyxoviruses while influenza is classified as orthomyxovirus. The influenza viruses are usually associated with epidemic respiratory disease in all age groups, whereas the parainfluenza viruses are usually associated with endemic respiratory infection in children.

Members of the myxovirus group are single-stranded RNA viruses; each virus particle consists of a nucleoprotein helix surrounded by a lipoprotein envelope. The influenza virus contains an 8-segmented single-stranded RNA genome enclosed in an envelope about 100 nm in diameter (figure 40). The parainfluenza viruses are 150–300 nm in diameter (figures 41 and 42). Each has a large nonsegmented inner helix. Budding from the plasma membrane is seen in both influenza and parainfluenza virus–infected cells. Morphologic distinctions between the influenza virus and parainfluenza virus are easily recognized by electron microscopy (figures 40–42). Virus infectivity is readily destroyed by ether treatment and the particles are relatively heat-labile.

Free virus particles characteristically exhibit well-defined spikes, consisting of hemagglutinin and neuraminidase, on the envelopes. Their ability to adsorb onto the surface of red blood cells, the hemagglutination phenomenon, is a unique property of this group; erythrocyte agglutination occurs at 4°C or 22°C but not at 37°C (tables 4 and 17). Guinea pig RBC are preferable for testing of new influenza type A and B isolates, whereas day-old chicken RBC are more satisfactory for influenza type C hemagglutination.

Influenza and parainfluenza viruses are capable of multiplying in a variety of animals as well as in various tissue culture systems. In addition to primary monkey kidney cells, the GPE cells are highly susceptible to parainfluenza virus types 3 and 5. Since viruses in this group do not regularly induce extensive

Table 17. Properties of Influenza and Parainfluenza Viruses

| Virus Types | Host Systems | | Hemagglutination at Various Temperatures Using RBC Obtained from | | | | |
	Embryonated Eggs	Tissue Culture	Chick 4°C	Chick 22°C	Guinea Pig 4°C	Guinea Pig 22°C	Human (type O) 22°C
Orthomyxovirus							
Influenza							
A	+	+/−	+	+	+	+	+
B	+	+	+	+	+	+	+
C	+	−	+	−	−	−	−
Paramyxovirus							
Parainfluenza							
1(HA-2)	+	+	+	+	+	+	+
2(CA)	−	+	+	+	+	+	+
3(HA-1)	−	+	+	+	+	+	+
4(M-25)	−	+	−	−	+	+	+
5(SV$_5$-SA-DA)	+/−	+	+	+	+	+	+
Mumps	+	+/−	+	+	+	+	+
NDV	+	+	+	+	+	+	+

Key: + = virus-induced change
− = no change

CPE, the *hemadsorption* technique is used to recognize their presence in tissue culture (see below). The presence of only minimum CPE during virus multiplication may be due to the action of protective inhibitor substances produced as the result of cell infection. Such an inhibitor or interferon was originally described by Isaacs and Lindeman in the influenza virus–infected chick embryo cell system.

Specimen Inoculation

Throat washings and throat or nasopharyngeal swabs are used for isolation of influenza and parainfluenza viruses. Tissues collected at autopsy, especially lungs, can be used for influenza virus isolation. Embryonated chicken eggs, 10 to 11 days old, are the simplest and most widely used host system for the recovery of influenza virus isolates (for egg inoculation procedure, see chapter 3). Primary monkey kidney cell cultures are the most sensitive cell system for the isolation of the parainfluenza viruses, although certain strains of influenza virus have been isolated in tissue culture. It is advisable that culture medium contain no serum. For example, culture medium in the absence of calf serum, lactalbumin hydrolysate, and maintained at pH 6.8 is a favorable medium for the multiplication of myxoviruses. Incubation at 33°C is more favorable than at

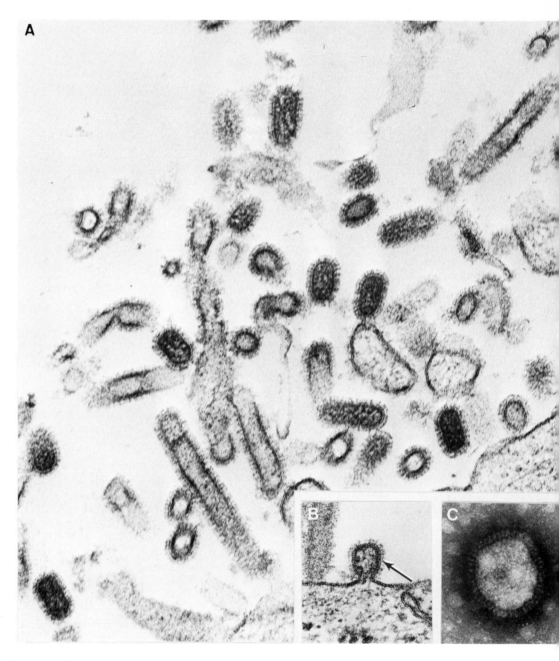

Figure 40. A. Electron micrograph of an influenza virus A2/Tex/78–infected monkey kidney cell,
showing virus particles at the extracellular space (100,800X).
B. Virus particle budding at the cell membrane (100,800X).
C. Influenza virus particle stained with PTA (168,000X).

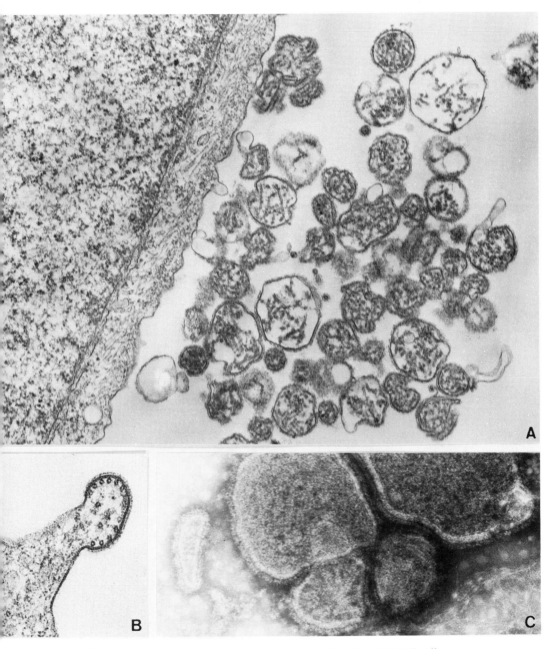

Figure 41. Electron micrographs of a parainfluenza virus type 3–infected RhMK cell.
    A. Thin section of an infected cell, showing many extracellular virus particles (38,400X).
    B. A virus particle in the process of budding at the cell membrane (70,400X).
    C. Virus particles negatively stained with PTA (100,800X).

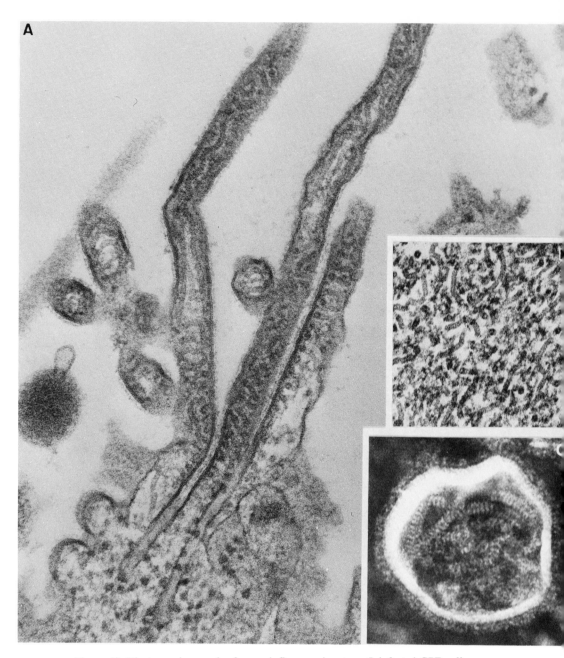

Figure 42. Electron micrograph of a parainfluenza virus type 5–infected GPE cell.
 A. Filamentous-form virus particles (SV$_5$) budding at a cell surface (100,800X) (courtesy of F. Bia).
 B. Helical viral nucleocapsids in the cytoplasm (79,200X).
 C. Virus particle (DA), negatively stained with PTA revealing internal nucleocapsid structure (126,150X) (courtesy of J. D. Wright).

142

37°C. A canine kidney cell line, MDCK, has been found highly sensitive for the isolation of influenza virus when the medium contained trypsin-EDTA solution (2 μg/ml trypsin and 0.9 μg/ml ethylene-diamine tetraacetic acid).

Virus Isolation, Propagation, and Assay

Hemadsorption in cell cultures. Ordinarily, influenza and parainfluenza virus–infected cell cultures do not exhibit any distinctive cellular changes. However, when a freshly obtained guinea pig RBC suspension is added to the infected cultures, the RBC adsorb onto the infected cells, resulting in the hemadsorption phenomenon as shown in figure 43. When a culture shows positive hemadsorption, the culture fluid is subcultured into a fresh culture to confirm the virus isolation and to permit further identification. However, caution should be taken when aged guinea pig RBC are used, since nonspecific hemadsorption often occurs in an uninoculated culture (figure 44) and should be distinguished from that resulting from a specific viral infection. Furthermore, hemadsorption usually takes place at 4°C or 22°C since the RBC will elute when incubated at 37°C. The technique is as follows:

1. Remove fluids from the inoculated cultures and collect in a sterile tube, then add 0.2 ml of the 0.5% guinea pig RBC suspension to each inoculated culture.
2. Place tubes in refrigerator at 4°C in a horizontal position for 20 minutes; make sure that the RBC suspension is in contact with the infected cells.
3. Remove unadsorbed RBC by washing the culture with cold PBS.
4. Read the tubes microscopically for hemadsorption, and record the results as −, +, + +, + + +, + + + +, according to the concentration of adsorbed RBC. An example of a positive hemadsorption is shown in figure 43.
5. Subculture the fluid from the culture showing hemadsorption into fresh cultures for further identification.
6. Nonspecific hemadsorption often occurs in the uninfected control cultures when aged guinea pig RBC are used (figure 44) and should be distinguished from that resulting from specific viral infection.

Certain strains of parainfluenza virus, particularly parainfluenza 3, produce multinucleated syncytial cells in infected Hep-2 or HeLa cells, as shown in figure 45. These cultures will also exhibit hemadsorption when a guinea pig RBC suspension is added. Some strains of influenza virus, especially influenza B, may produce some cellular changes in infected cultures. The infected cells become progressively granular, swollen, and round; later they become pycnotic and fragmented, and finally the whole cell sheet is destroyed. Again, when guinea pig RBC are added hemadsorption also occurs.

Embryonated egg inoculation. Most of the influenza A virus strains propagate best in embryonated eggs. For primary isolation, specimens should be inoculated by the amniotic route (see chapter 3). Inoculated eggs are candled

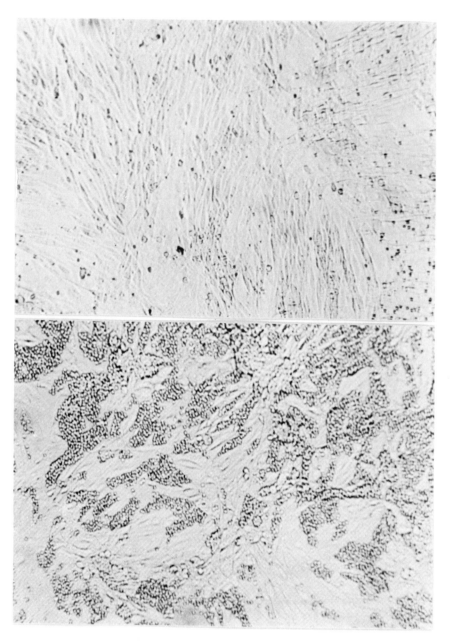

Figure 43. Hemadsorption of a myxovirus-infected RhMK culture (100X). Upper: Uninoculated RhMK culture. Lower: RhMK culture infected with parainfluenza virus type 1, showing hemadsorption of guinea pig erythrocytes.

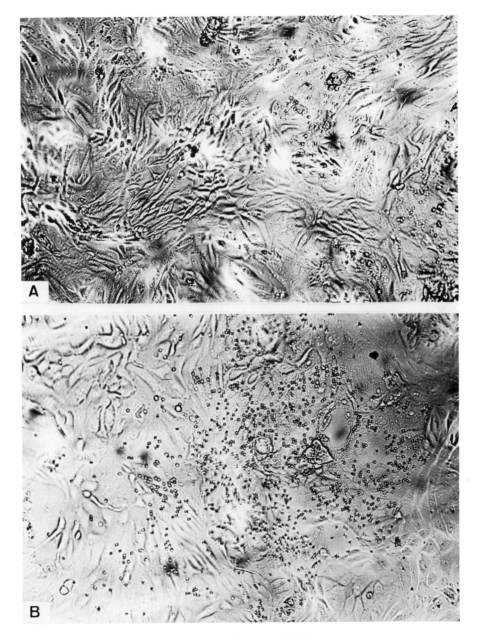

Figure 44. Nonspecific hemadsorption in RhMK culture (100X).
A. Uninfected RhMK culture.
B. Nonspecific hemadsorption resulting when aged guinea pig RBC were used (compare with figure 43).

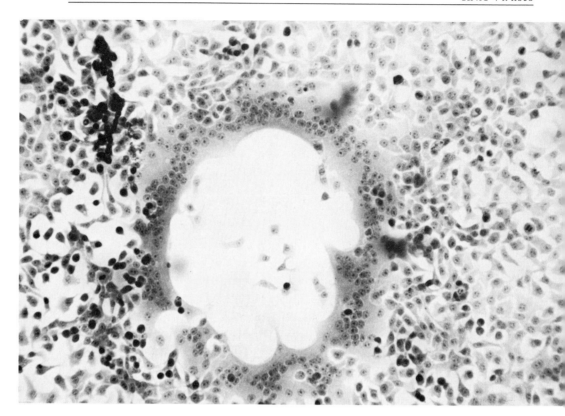

Figure 45. Syncytial cell formation induced by parainfluenza virus type 3 in Hep-2 cell culture 3 days after infection (H&E, 100X).

daily. Embryos that die within 24 hours of inoculation are discarded. Egg fluids are harvested 2 to 3 days after influenza virus inoculation. Both allantoic fluid (ALF) and amniotic fluid (AMF) can be aspirated from the infected eggs with a capillary pipette. The egg fluids are tested for hemagglutinin with 0.5% guinea pig RBC suspension. It is important to chill embryos prior to harvesting the egg fluids to prevent bleeding from the chorioallantoic vessels when the membrane is cut and removed. Excessive bleeding may result in loss of virus due to attachment of viral particles to RBC.

Plaque formation and interference phenomenon. Even though the plaque technique is not routinely used for primary isolation of influenza and parainfluenza viruses, plaque formation has been used to assay virus infectivity titers especially for strains of parainfluenza viruses. In order to demonstrate virus plaques, serial 10-fold dilutions of culture fluids should be made so as to obviate the effect of any interference that may be produced when a large virus inoculum is used. Autoinhibition and restriction of plaque development have been observed with certain parainfluenza viruses, as illustrated in figure 46.

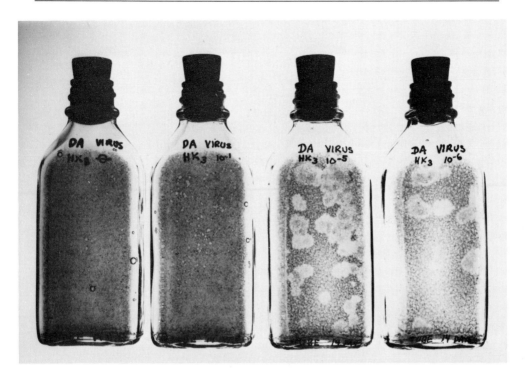

Figure 46. Autoinhibition of plaque formation by a myxovirus inhibitor (G. D. Hsiung et al., *J. Immunol*. 88: 284, 1962). Two bottles at left were inoculated with parainfluenza virus type 5 (DA)–infected tissue culture fluid, undiluted and 10^{-1}; no evidence of virus plaque. Two bottles at right were inoculated with 10^{-5} and 10^{-6} of the same virus suspension; virus-induced plaques are clearly visible.

Identification of Isolates

Complement-fixation and hemagglutination-inhibition tests. Most of the influenza viruses isolated in embryonated eggs can be identified by the CF test against known group-specific antiserum (for CF test procedure, see chapter 6) and by the HI test for virus type or strain identification (for HI test procedure, see chapter 5). In the HI test both ALF and AMF can be used as HA antigens and can be tested against known type-specific influenza virus antiserum. Upon initial isolation of influenza virus in eggs, the AMF often yields higher titers of HA antigen than the ALF. Guinea pig erythrocytes in PBS should be used for the HA or HI tests since chick erythrocytes are often not agglutinable with primary isolates of influenza A viruses. It should be noted that nonspecific inhibitors may be present in many animal sera, thus interfering with the identification procedure. (For removal of nonspecific inhibitors, see p. 40.)

Hemadsorption-inhibition method. The parainfluenza viruses are routinely identified by the hemadsorption-inhibition test in tissue culture systems as described below. Some strains of influenza virus when grown in cell culture can also be identified by the hemadsorption-inhibition test.

1. Inoculate serial 10-fold dilutions of the virus suspension into tissue culture tubes. After 3–5 days, test for hemadsorption with guinea pig erythrocytes. Calculate the $TCID_{50}$ end point.
2. Prepare 2-, 4-, or 10-fold dilutions of antiserum (all sera should be heat-inactivated at 56°C for 30 minutes).
3. Add an equal volume of a constant dilution of the unknown virus containing 30 to 50 $TCID_{50}$ (50% hemadsorption tissue culture dose, in this instance) to each of the serum dilutions; mix well.
4. Allow the virus-serum mixtures and the control test virus suspension to remain at room temperature for 1 hour.
5. Inoculate 0.2 ml amounts of the virus-serum mixtures into culture tubes, using 3 or 4 tubes for each serum dilution.
6. For the virus control, inoculate 0.1 ml of the serial 10-fold dilutions of the virus suspension into each tube, using 3 or 4 tubes per dilution.
7. Test all cultures for hemadsorption 3–5 days after inoculation by adding 0.2 ml of a 0.5% freshly obtained guinea pig RBC suspension to each tube. Refrigerate for 20 minutes and read. (It is advisable to test the virus control tubes inoculated with 30–50 $TCID_{50}$ *first*; if hemadsorption is observed in these challenge virus tubes, all other tubes are ready for testing.)
8. Complete inhibition of hemadsorption by a known antiserum is considered a positive serum neutralization test and indicates the identity of the virus. The serum titer is the highest dilution inhibiting multiplication of the challenge virus so that no hemadsorption is detected.

Serodiagnosis

Serologic tests have been used for detection and/or diagnosis of influenza virus infections, particularly in suspected cases. Diagnosis of influenza may be made when a significant antibody rise is observed to the internal antigens, the "S" antigen consisting of membrane protein and nucleoprotein or the surface "V" antigens consisting of hemagglutinin and neuraminidase. The "S" antigens are group-specific and antigenically stable. The CF test is most frequently used for determination of serum antibody to the "S" antigens, which are common to the same influenza group, but antibody rises to purified "V" antigens are indicative of a specific virus strain.

In the HI test for influenza virus, it is necessary to destroy the nonspecific inhibitors present in the serum. Receptor-destroying enzyme (RDE) is used to remove inhibitors in human and chick serum (see chapter 5), Kaolin treatment is used for guinea pig serum, and trypsin and periodate treatment is used for inhibitors present in equine serum. The procedures for CF and HI tests are described in chapters 5 and 6.

Isolating Mumps Virus from Urine

Direct Inoculation

1. Remove fluid from primary monkey kidney cell culture tubes and inoculate undiluted freshly obtained urine directly into each culture, 0.3 to 0.5 ml per tube. (Seven- to 8-day-old embryonated eggs may also be used.)
2. Adsorb for 2 hours at 37°C.
3. Drain urine from the inoculated cultures and replace with fresh medium.
4. For egg inoculation procedure, see chapter 3.

Concentration Method

1. Centrifuge 15 ml urine at 500 × g at 4°C for 10 minutes.
2. Collect 10 ml of the supernatant and recentrifuge at 100,000 × g for 90 minutes in an ultracentrifuge.
3. Resuspend the pellet in 1.0 ml of Hanks' BSS and inoculate into culture tubes (or embryonated eggs), 0.1 to 0.2 ml per tube (or per egg).

Test for Result

With inoculated cultures, check CPE and test for hemadsorption 7 to 10 days after inoculation. For inoculated embryonated eggs, harvest AMF and ALF 5–7 days after inoculation and test for hemagglutinin in the egg fluids as described above for the influenza virus.

Mumps virus isolation procedures are not routinely done because of the slow growth rate of the virus; therefore serodiagnosis has been commonly performed. A significant antibody rise by CF or HI method is an indication of mumps virus infection.

SUPPLEMENTARY READING

Books and Review Papers

Chanock, R. M. Parainfluenza viruses. In *Diagnostic procedures for viral, rickettsial and chlamydial infections*, ed. E. H. Lennette and N. J. Schmidt, p. 611. 5th ed. Washington, D.C.: American Public Health Association, 1979.

Choppin, P. W., and Compans, R. W. Reproduction of paramyxoviruses. *Compar. Virology* 4: 95, 1975.

Dowdle, W. A., Kendal, A. P., and Noble, G. R. Influenza viruses. In *Diagnostic procedures for viral, rickettsial and chlamydial infections,* ed. E. H. Lennette and N. J. Schmidt, p. 585. 5th ed. Washington, D.C.: American Public Health Association, 1979.

Hsiung, G. D. Parainfluenza 5 virus infection of man and animals. *Progr. Med. Virol.* 14: 241, 1972.

Kilbourne, E. D. The influenza viruses and influenza. New York: Academic Press, 1975.

Specific Articles

Daisy, J. A. Rapid diagnosis of influenza A infection by direct immunofluorescence of nasopharyngeal aspirates in adults. *J. Clin. Micro.* 9: 688, 1979.

Dowdle, W. R., and Robinson, R. Q. Non-specific hemadsorption by rhesus monkey kidney cells. *Proc. Soc. Exp. Biol. Med.* 121: 193, 1966.

Frank, A. L., Couch, R. B., Griffis, C. A., and Baxter, B. D. Comparison of different tissue cultures for isolation and quantitation of influenza and parainfluenza viruses. *J. Clin. Micro.* 10: 32, 1979.

Hawthorne, J. D., and Albrecht, P. Sensitive plaque neutralization assay for parainfluenza virus types 1, 2, and 3 and respiratory virus. *J. Clin. Micro.* 13: 730, 1981.

Hirst, G. K. The agglutination of red cells by allantoic fluid of chick embryos infected with influenza virus. *Science* 94: 22, 1941.

Monto, A. S., Moassab, H. F., and Bryan, E. R. Relative efficacy of embryonated eggs and cell culture for isolation of contemporary influenza viruses. *J. Clin. Micro.* 13: 233, 1981.

Palese, P., and Schulman, J. L. Mapping of the influenza virus genome: identification of the hemagglutination and the neuraminidase genes. *Proc. Natl. Acad. Sci. U.S.A.* 73: 2142, 1976.

Parkinson, A. J., Muchmore, H. G., Scott, L. V., and Miles, J. A. Parainfluenza virus isolation enhancement utilizing a portable cell culture system in the field. *J. Clin. Micro.* 11: 535, 1980.

16. Pseudomyxoviridae

Measles and respiratory syncytial viruses resemble the parainfluenza viruses morphologically but biologically and serologically are distinctly different (table 18). These two viruses are similar in size and shape to the parainfluenza viruses. Although measles virus hemagglutinates monkey erythrocytes, hemagglutinin has not been described for respiratory syncytial virus. Furthermore, no neuraminidase can be detected in the measles virus. Thus, the name pseudomyxovirus has been proposed for these agents; however, it has not yet been accepted for use in any classification scheme.

MEASLES VIRUS

Measles is an exanthematous disease that has a high morbidity rate in young children. The virus can be isolated from throat washings and blood of patients if specimens are collected not later than the first 24 hours after the appearance of a rash. Since isolation is difficult and time-consuming, in doubtful cases serologic tests, either CF or HI, are more useful than virus isolation in establishing a diagnosis.

Like the parainfluenza viruses, the measles virus is a single-stranded RNA virus, consisting of a nucleoprotein helix enclosed by a lipoprotein envelope (figure 47). The size of the measles virus particle ranges from 150 to 300 nm. Virus infectivity is inactivated by ether. The infectious virus is relatively unstable with respect to temperature and to pH below 5 or above 10.

Measles virus can be cultivated in a variety of primate and nonprimate cells. Characteristic multinucleated giant cells are observed in infected cultures both in MK and serial cell lines. Although measles virus–infected cell culture fluids contain hemagglutinin and react with erythrocytes from simian primates, including patas and green monkeys, they do not agglutinate nonsimian RBC, including human cells; this characteristic is useful for separating measles virus from other

Table 18. Properties of Measles and Respiratory Syncytial Viruses

Virus Type	Cell Culture System	CPE	Eosinophilic Inclusion	Hemagglutination in Tissue Culture Fluid	Identification Method of Choice
Measles	MK & HEK	multi-nucleated syncytial cells	intracyto-plasmic and intranuclear	$+^a$	HI, CF, NT
	Hep-2	syncytial cells	−	+	
Respiratory Syncytial	Hep-2	multi-nucleated syncytial cells	occasionally intra-cytoplasmic	−	IF, CF, NT
	GM–BSC-1	multi-nucleated		−	
	A549	syncytial cells	+	−	

^{a}Monkey erythrocytes only; no enzymatic reaction can be detected.

Key: + = virus-induced change
        − = no change

paramyxovirus types. In hematoxylin-eosin-stained preparations of primary MK or HEK cultures infected with measles virus, eosinophilic intranuclear and intra-cytoplasmic inclusions are easily seen. Measles virus induces characteristic multinucleated giant cells in Hep-2 cell cultures, including cells in mitosis, but no intranuclear inclusions are found in the latter.

Specimen Inoculation

Whole blood or buffy coat, throat washings, and urine have been used for virus isolation. Primary monkey kidney cells and human embryonic kidney cell cultures are the most susceptible host systems, although laboratory strains can grow in the Hep-2 cell line.

Acute and convalescent sera are used for serodiagnostic purposes.

Virus Isolation, Propagation, and Assay

Cytopathic effect in fluid cultures. Measles virus induces typical foamy-like cellular changes in primary human kidney or MK cell cultures (figure 48B).

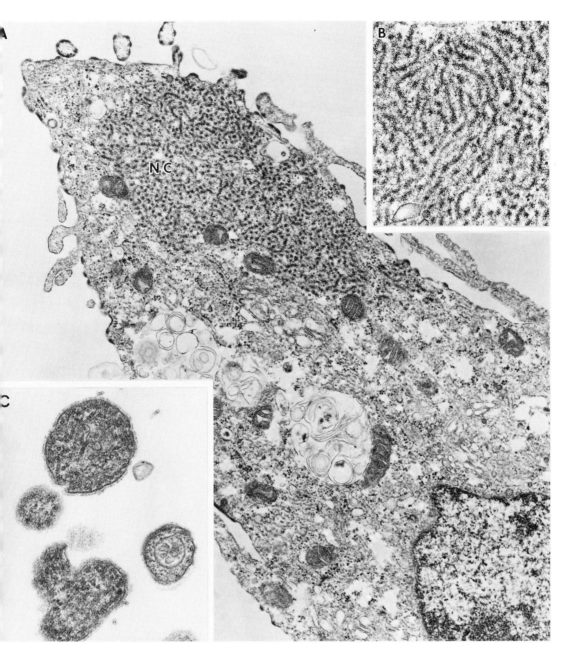

Figure 47. Electron micrograph of a measles virus–infected Vero cell.
    A. Measles virus inclusion containing helical nucleocapsids (NC) in the cytoplasm
       (19,680X).
    B. High magnification of viral nucleocapsids (30,000X).
    C. Measles virus particles in the extracellular space (48,000X).

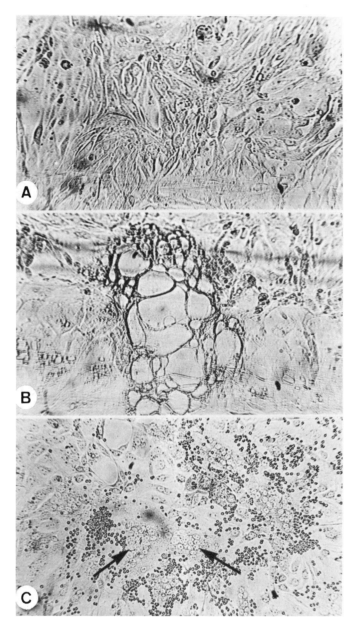

Figure 48. Syncytial cell formation and hemadsorption of measles virus–infected RhMK cell cultures (100X).
A. Uninfected RhMK culture.
B. Foamy appearance of CPE caused by measles virus.
C. Multinucleated cells (arrows) and hemadsorption of monkey RBC induced by measles virus.

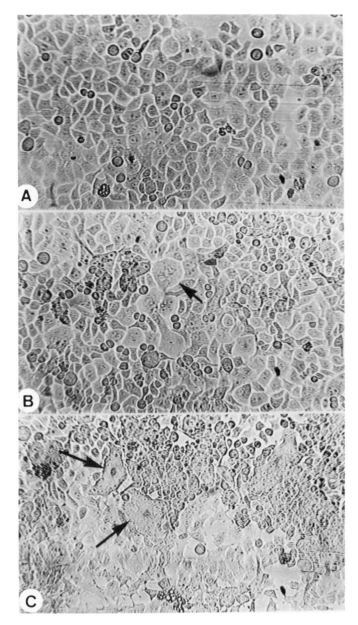

Figure 49. Syncytial cell formation induced by measles virus in Hep-2 cell cultures (100X).
    A. Uninfected Hep-2 cell culture.
    B. Early appearance of multinucleated cells (arrow).
    C. Advanced appearance of multinucleated cells (arrow).

Human embryonic kidney cultures are apparently the most suitable system for primary virus isolation. Cultures should be maintained as long as possible, for 4 to 6 weeks, with frequent changes of medium. It is also advisable to transfer infected culture fluids, diluted 1:10, to fresh culture tubes at weekly intervals, carrying them through several blind passages before a negative result is reported. After laboratory adaptation, measles virus also replicates in Hep-2 cultures, producing multinucleated syncytial cells (figure 49).

Whole blood specimens from which virus isolation attempts are to be made should be processed immediately or stored in the refrigerator and processed within six hours:

1. Centrifuge heparinized blood for 20 minutes at 500 × g.
2. Remove plasma and resuspend cells in Hanks' BSS to the original volume.
3. Inoculate 0.5-ml amounts of the blood cell suspension into three or more tubes of human kidney cell cultures. (Since measles virus is usually associated with leukocytes, the latter are good sources for virus isolation.)
4. After 24–48 hours' incubation at 37°C, but no later than the third day, wash the cultures with 3 changes of medium and replace with fresh medium.
5. Observe cultures intermittently for cytopathic changes, for 4–6 weeks, replacing the maintenance medium three times a week.

Hemadsorption in cell cultures. Measles virus–infected cells show hemadsorption upon the addition of 0.5% monkey RBC (figure 48C). Since guinea pig and human RBC are not similarly hemadsorbed, this reaction provides a useful indicator that the cultures are infected with the measles and not another paramyxovirus.

Cytopathology in measles virus–infected cells. Measles virus induces characteristic intranuclear and intracytoplasmic eosinophilic inclusions in infected primary monkey or human kidney cells (figure 50). These can be demonstrated when infected cells are fixed and stained with hematoxylin-eosin.

Plaque formation under agar overlay. Measles virus produces distinct pinpoint plaques in primary monkey kidney cell cultures (figure 51). Although this method is not used for routine isolation purposes, it can be used for quantitative assay of measles virus.

Identification of Isolates

Neutralization test in tissue culture. The test can be set up in primary HEK cultures or in Hep-2 tube cultures with 100 $TCID_{50}$ as the challenge dose against known antiserum. Since measles CPE appears slowly, there is a direct relationship between the dilution of virus and the degeneration time of cells in culture. Thus the observation period should range from 2 to 3 weeks, especially when doses of less than 100 $TCID_{50}$ are used. Since CPE usually develops very slowly, the more sensitive hemadsorption-inhibition method described in the myxovirus

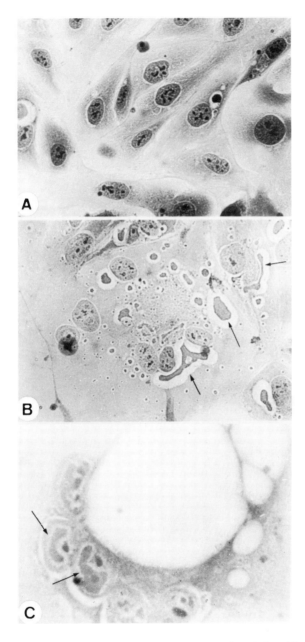

Figure 50. Eosinophilic intracytoplasmic and intranuclear inclusions induced by measles virus in HEK cell cultures (H&E).
  A. Uninfected HEK cell culture (400X).
  B. Intracytoplasmic inclusions (arrows) induced by measles virus (400X).
  C. Intranuclear inclusions (arrows) induced by measles virus (970X).

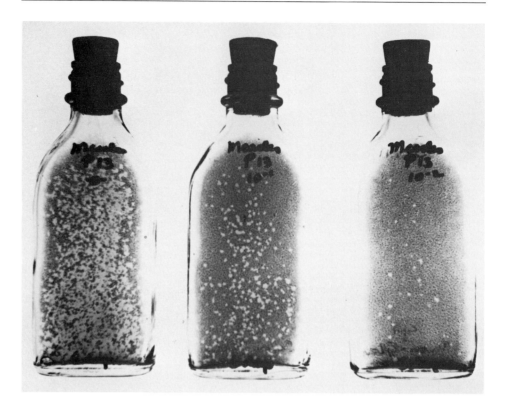

Figure 51. Plaque assay of measles virus in primary patas MK cell cultures, 6 days after inoculation (G. D. Hsiung, *Proc. Soc. Exp. Biol. Med.* 98: 68, 1958).

chapter (see p. 147) and the plaque-reduction neutralization method (see chapter 4) should be used for identification of measles virus isolates.

Hemagglutination, hemagglutination-inhibition, and hemolysin production by measles virus. Since the hemagglutinin (HA) titer in measles virus–infected cultures is often low, several methods have been used to concentrate the antigen in order to yield a sufficiently high titer of HA. Monkey erythrocytes, preferably from African green monkeys, resuspended to 0.5% in saline are used for the measles virus HA titrations. The cells are allowed to settle at 37°C for 1 hour. If hemagglutination of measles virus is observed, the HI test can be used for final identification of the virus. Provided the HA antigen is sufficiently potent, further incubation at 37°C for 4 hours may demonstrate specific hemolysin (for HA and HI procedures, see chapter 5).

Electron microscopy. The association of measles virus with subacute sclerosing panencephalitis (SSPE) was recognized through visualization of viral nucleocapsids with characteristic measles virus morphology in brain biopsy materials following thin sectioning. Electron microscopic examination of measles virus–infected cells reveals intranuclear and intracytoplasmic viral nucleocapsids (figure 47) that correspond to the viral inclusions seen by light microscopy. Extracellular virus particles can be seen occasionally (figure 47 inset).

Serodiagnosis

Hemagglutination-inhibition test. Although HI, CF, and neutralization tests are used for determination of measles virus infection, the HI test is the preferred method for measuring specific antibody.

Since human serum contains natural agglutinins for monkey RBC, the human sera being tested must be adsorbed with 50% monkey RBC in saline at 4°C overnight before use. The sera should also undergo kaolin treatment. Virus-serum mixtures are incubated at room temperature for 1 hour before the addition of monkey RBC, 0.5% in saline. For more sensitive results, the mixtures are incubated at 37°C for 1 hour after the addition of RBC. (For HI procedure, see chapter 5).

Complement-fixation test. Measles virus CF antigen can be prepared following propagation of measles virus in one of several cell lines. The following procedure using Hep-2 cells has been found satisfactory. Monolayer cultures, infected with measles virus, are harvested when cytopathic effects have progressed to a stage where the cells may be easily dislodged from the glass upon gentle shaking. The virus suspension obtained can then be quick-frozen in an alcohol–dry ice bath for subsequent storage at − 70°C. Measles virus pools may be anticomplementary, in which case heating at 56°C for 1 hour is recommended (for CF procedure, see chapter 6).

Neutralization tests either by inhibition of hemadsorption in Hep-2 cells or plaque reduction in Hep-2 bottle cultures have been used. Although they are sensitive and reliable tests, the waiting period for results is usually 2 weeks.

RESPIRATORY SYNCYTIAL VIRUS

Respiratory syncytial virus (RSV) has been associated chiefly with respiratory illness in children; it occasionally affects adults. The virus is present in the upper respiratory tract early in the course of the illness and has been recovered from nasal or throat swabs or washings as long as 7 to 8 days after onset. It is extremely labile and poorly withstands freezing and thawing. Specimens for virus isolation should therefore be inoculated directly into tissue cultures when received by the laboratory.

RSV is a pleomorphic virus, spherical and with a diameter of 150 to 300 nm, similar to the measles virus (figure 52). It does not multiply in embryonated eggs but grows in cell cultures of a variety of animal species as well as in several cell lines, including A549, Hep-2, and HeLa. The virus envelope surrounds the helical nucleocapsid. In tissue culture the virus produces character-

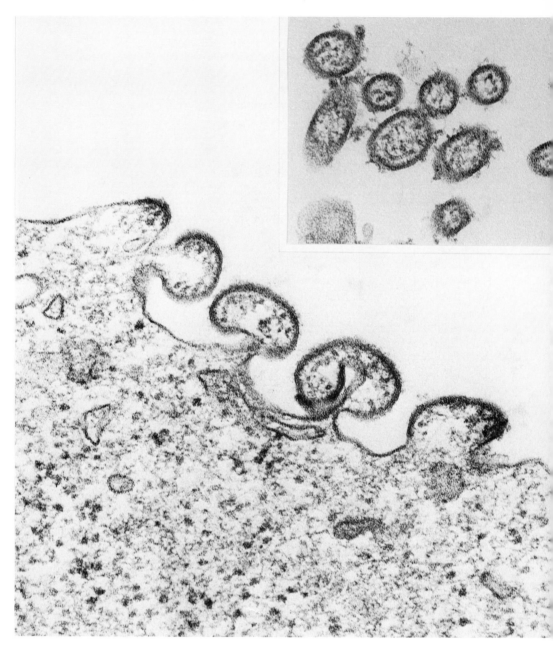

Figure 52. Electron micrograph of respiratory syncytial virus (RSV) in an A549 cell, showing several virus particles in the process of budding at the cell membrane (100,800X). Inset: cross section of extracellular virus particles (100,800X).

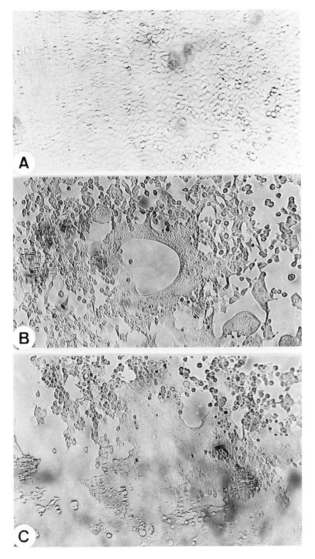

Figure 53. Syncytial cell formation induced by RSV in Hep-2 cell cultures (100X).
    A. Uninoculated cell control.
    B. RSV-infected cells at 3 days.
    C. RSV-infected cells at 5 days.

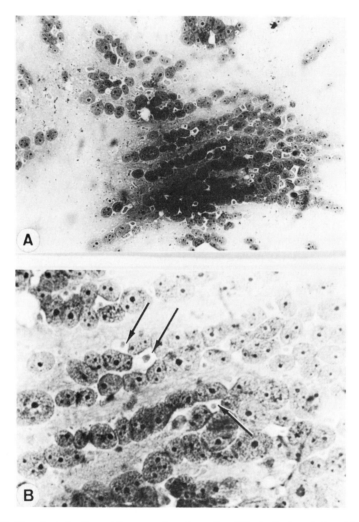

Figure 54. Multinucleated cells and intracytoplasmic eosinophilic inclusions induced by RSV in
BSC-1 green MK cell line culture (H&E).
A. Multinucleated cells (100X).
B. Intracytoplasmic inclusions (arrows) (400X).

istic syncytial cells (figure 53), from which its name is derived. No hemagglutinin or neuraminidase activity has yet been discovered. Stained preparations of infected cells reveal eosinophilic intracytoplasmic inclusions (figure 54).

Methods for isolation and identification are similar to those described for measles virus except that Hep-2 and now A549 cell cultures are the most sensitive systems for RSV isolation; the characteristic syncytial formation is most easily detected in them. RSV can be identified by the immunofluorescent staining technique using known antiserum to the virus (for procedure, see chapter 9). Final identification of the virus can be made by the neutralization test in tissue culture or by the CF test. An ELISA has been developed for the detection of serum antibody against RSV. Antibody titers detected by the ELISA are 100 times higher than those tested by CF and 2–4 times higher than the plaque-reduction neutralization test.

SUPPLEMENTARY READING

Measles Virus

Books and Review Papers

Black, F. L. Measles. In *Viral infections of humans, epidemiology and control,* ed. A. S. Evans, p. 297. New York: Plenum Medical Books, 1976.

Morgan, E. M., and Rapp, F. Measles virus and its associated diseases. *Bact. Rev.* 41: 636, 1977.

Olding-Stenkvist, E., Bjorvatn, E. Rapid detection of measles virus in skin rashes by immunofluorescence. *J. Infect. Dis.* 134: 463, 1976.

Specific Articles

Kleiman, M. B., Blackburn, C. K. L., Zimmerman, S. E., and French, M. L. V. Comparison of enzyme-linked immunosorbent assay for acute measles with hemagglutination inhibition, complement-fixation, and fluorescent antibody methods. *J. Clin. Micro.* 14: 147, 1981.

Norrby, E., Ruckle, G. E., and Meulen, V. T. Differences in the appearance of antibodies to structural components of measles virus after immunization with inactivated and live virus. *J. Infect. Dis.* 132: 262, 1975.

Respiratory Syncytial Viruses

Specific Articles

Chao, R. K., Fishaut, M., Schwartzman, J. D., and McIntosh, K. Detection of respiratory syncytial virus in nasal secretions from infants by enzyme-linked immunosorbent assay. *J. Infect. Dis.* 139: 483, 1979.

Gardner, P. S., McQuillin, J., and McGuskin, R. The late detection of respiratory syncytial virus in cells of respiratory tract by immunofluorescence. *J. Hyg.* 68: 575, 1970.

Hall, C. B., and Douglas, R. G., Jr. Clinically useful method for the isolation of respiratory syncytial virus. *J. Infect. Dis.* 131: 1, 1975.

Kaul, T. N., Welliver, R. C., and Ogra, P. L. Comparison of fluorescent-antibody, neutralizing-antibody, and complement-enhanced neutralizing antibody assays for detection of serum antibody to respiratory syncytial virus. *J. Clin. Micro.* 13: 957, 1981.

Marquez, A., and Hsiung, G. D. Influence of glutamine on multiplication and cytopathic effect of respiratory syncytial virus. *Proc. Soc. Exp. Biol. and Med.* 124: 95, 1967.

Richardson, L. S., Yolken, R. H., Belshe, R. B., Camargo, E., Kim, H. W., and Chanock, R. M. Enzyme-linked immunosorbent assay (ELISA) for measurement of serologic response to respiratory syncytial virus infection. *Inf. and Immun.* 20: 660, 1978.

17. Reoviridae

REOVIRUSES

Reoviruses occur widely in humans and a variety of animal species. Early reovirus isolates obtained from the stools of healthy children were identified collectively as echovirus type 10. They have been isolated occasionally from individuals with a variety of respiratory and enteric illnesses as well as from apparently healthy children. At present their role in human disease is not clear. The reoviruses, like the enterovirus group, are common inhabitants of the human intestinal tract and can be recovered from fecal specimens but infrequently from throat swabs.

Reovirus particles are approximately 70 nm in diameter (figure 55), icosahedral in shape, with a double-layer capsid; each consists of 92 capsomeres and a double-stranded RNA core with 10–12 segments. Since this is the first group of animal viruses shown to possess a double-stranded RNA genome, reoviruses have been studied more intensively by the molecular virologists than by those concerned with human disease. Viruses of this group are ether-resistant and relatively stable but vary in their pathogenicity for suckling mice.

Unlike enteroviruses, reoviruses are capable of multiplying and inducing CPE in a variety of nonprimate cells derived from pig, calf, dog, cat, guinea pig, and hamster. Serologically, they may be divided into three antigenic groups based upon neutralization and hemagglutination-inhibition reactions; all reoviruses share a common group complement-fixing antigen. Reovirus types 1 and 2 agglutinate human type-O erythrocytes at high titers whereas agglutination by type 3 is best with bovine erythrocytes at 4°C. Thus, differentiation of type 3 from types 1 and 2 may be made on this basis (see table 19).

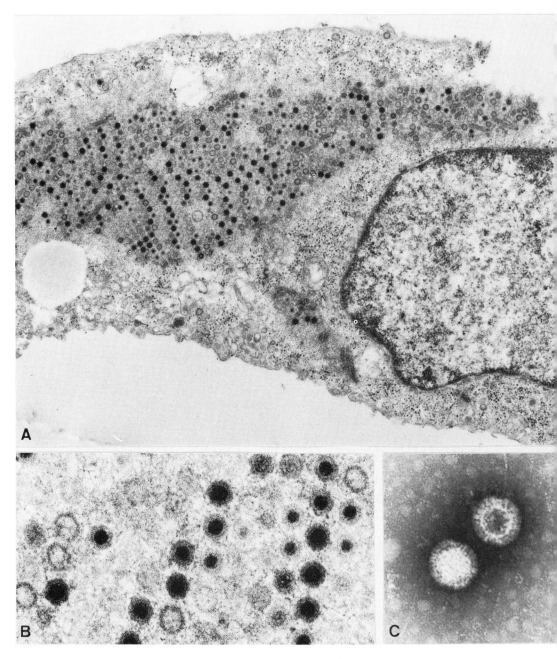

Figure 55. Electron micrographs of reovirus in RhMK cell.
      A. Thin section of reovirus type 1–infected RhMK cell, showing a large viral aggregate containing many virus particles in the cytoplasm (19,680X) (C. K. Y. Fong and G. D. Hsiung, in *Virology and rickettsiology* vol. 1, pt. 1, p. 62).
      B. Higher magnification of virus particles shown in A (88,000X).
      C. Reovirus particles stained with PTA (168,000X).

Table 19. Hemagglutination Properties of Reoviruses

Serotype	Source of Virus Isolation	Hemagglutination with RBC		
		Human (type O)	Bovine	Guinea Pig
1	man, calf, monkey	+	−	−
2	man, chimpanzee, calf, monkey	+	−	−
3	man, calf, mouse	P[a]	+	−

[a]Partial hemagglutination or low hemagglutinin titer.

Key: + = virus induced change
− = no change

Specimen Inoculation

Stools, rectal swabs, and occasionally throat swabs are used for virus isolation. Primary kidney cell cultures of both primates and nonprimates are highly susceptible to infection with reoviruses.

Virus Isolation, Propagation, and Assay

Cytopathic effect in fluid cultures. The cytopathic effects produced by the reoviruses show cellular granulation, but not the characteristic rounding up of cells associated with enterovirus cytopathology; recognition of their presence requires some experience, since typical reovirus CPE may be confused with nonspecific cellular degeneration of aging cultures. Infected cells do not dislodge readily from the monolayer. Confirmation of the specificity of the cellular changes may be obtained by reproducing them after passage into other culture types, especially those derived from certain nonprimate species. Figure 56 illustrates the CPE induced by reovirus type 1 in cat and guinea pig kidney cell cultures; CPE is usually more evident in the second passage but may not be readily apparent until the fourth or fifth passage.

Hemagglutination. Reovirus-infected cells commonly do not show hemadsorption upon the addition of human type-O erythrocytes; however, fluids from the same infected culture show significant hemagglutinin titers with human type-O RBC but not with guinea pig erythrocytes (see tables 4 and 19). Such agglutination occurs at 4°C, 22°C, and 37°C. For practical purposes a 0.75% suspension of human type-O RBC in 0.85% NaCl is satisfactory for agglutination of reovirus types 1 and 2, but bovine RBC are more suitable for reovirus type 3.

Plaque formation in bottle cultures. Reovirus produces plaques under agar overlay medium. Although this technique has not been used for primary isolation, the plaque method has been used exclusively for quantitative assays of reovirus infectivity. Since calf serum, which is used in the regular agar overlay

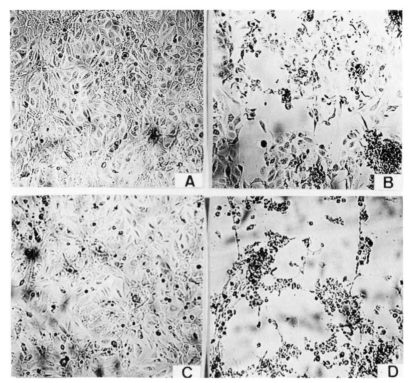

Figure 56. Cytopathic effect induced by reovirus in nonprimate kidney cell cultures (100X) (G. D. Hsiung, *Proc. Soc. Exp. Biol. Med.* 99: 387, 1958).
    A. Uninfected cat kidney cell culture, 17 days old.
    B. Cat kidney cell culture infected with reovirus type 1, 13 days after inoculation.
    C. Uninfected guinea pig kidney cell culture, 12 days old.
    D. Guinea pig kidney cell culture infected with reovirus type 1, 5 days after inoculation.

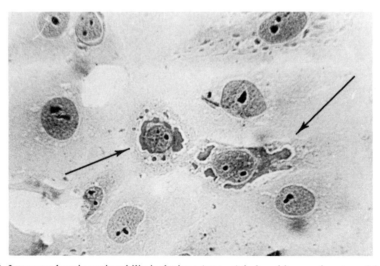

Figure 57. Intracytoplasmic eosinophilic inclusions (arrows) induced by reovirus type 1 in RhMK cells (H&E, 400X).

medium, may contain reovirus antibody, fetal bovine serum or skim milk provide satisfactory substitutes.

Cytopathology in immunofluorescent and H&E-stained preparations. Due to the unusual nonspecific appearance of CPE induced by the reoviruses, stained preparations are helpful for confirmation of the isolates. Characteristic reovirus intracytoplasmic eosinophilic inclusions in hematoxylin-eosin-stained preparations (figure 57 and color figure 3) are distinguishable from those produced by other groups of viruses. The presence of these perinuclear inclusions permits a presumptive diagnosis of a reovirus infection. These inclusions also can be easily recognized after infected cells are stained with acridine orange (see color figure 4). In the latter preparation the cytoplasmic yellowish green inclusions are characteristic of the double-stranded RNA reovirus. Brilliant fluorescent cytoplasmic inclusions are easily detected in infected cells by both direct and indirect immunofluorescent techniques (figures 58 and 59).

Identification of Isolates

Complement-fixation test. The three reovirus types share a group antigen that can be detected by the CF test, but this method cannot identify the individual serotypes.

Hemagglutination-inhibition test. The HI test is used for identification of specific reovirus serotypes. The typing sera should be treated with 25% kaolin in 0.85% NaCl. After kaolin treatment, the sera should be adsorbed with washed, packed human type-O erythrocytes to remove any natural agglutinins to the human RBC that are present in the sera. (Although procedures for the HI test are the same as described in chapter 5, note that 0.85% NaCl is used instead of PBS for the human type-O erythrocyte suspension and the RBCs are allowed to settle at 22°C for best results.)

Neutralization test. Inhibition of CPE or plaque-reduction neutralization test can be performed in rhesus monkey kidney cell cultures or guinea pig embryo cells using 100 $TCID_{50}$ as the challenge dose against type-specific antisera.

Electron microscopy. Reovirus particles have a distinctive morphology. It is fairly easy to recognize their presence using negatively stained virus preparations (figure 55 inset). In infected cells, reovirus develops characteristic intracytoplasmic inclusions. Electron microscopic examination of fixed and embedded cells reveals virus aggregates in the cytoplasm of infected cells (figure 55) corresponding to the inclusions seen by light microscopy (figure 57).

Serodiagnosis

Hemagglutination-inhibition test. The diagnosis of most reovirus infections has been determined through the HI test because of its simplicity and sensitivity as well as its specificity. All human sera should be heated at 56°C for 30 minutes and treated with kaolin before use, as described above, using the test procedure described in chapter 5.

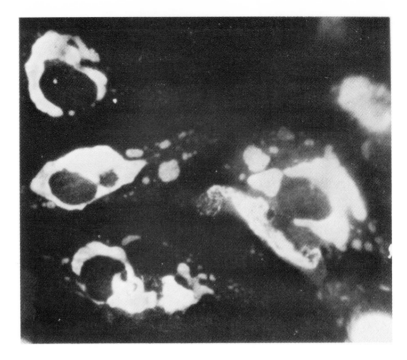

Figure 58. Intracytoplasmic inclusions induced by reovirus type 1 in RhMK cells 54 hours after infection (IF staining preparation, direct method, 540X). Note the brilliant fluorescent inclusions that surround the nuclei (J. S. Rhim et al., *Virology* 17: 342, 1962).

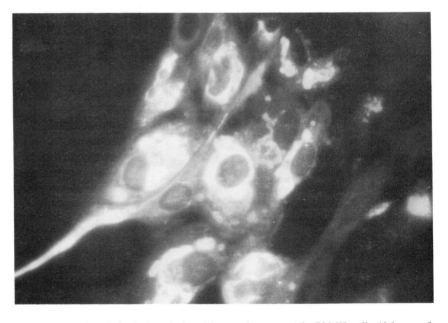

Figure 59. Intracytoplasmic inclusions induced by reovirus type 1 in RhMK cells 40 hours after infection (IF staining preparation, indirect method, 400X).

ROTAVIRUSES

Rotaviruses are a group of viruses that infect humans and a variety of nonhuman species; they cause acute diarrhea in infants, calves, piglets, newborn mice, etc. Prior to the 1970s, evidence for etiologic agents in cases of acute infectious nonbacterial gastroenteritis was inconclusive. In 1973, rotavirus particles were first observed in patients with gastroenteritis and, in 1974, reoviruslike agents were noted in stool samples obtained from patients with infantile diarrhea. Subsequently, rotavirus was designated as the causative agent associated with these diseases.

Morphologically, the rotavirus ("rota," from Latin "a wheel") exhibits a wheellike structure, 70–75 nm in diameter, with two capsid layers (figure 60). Rotavirus possesses 11-segmented double-stranded RNA genomes.

Although the rotavirus in stool is stable at room temperature for several months, propagation of the virus to high concentrations in cell cultures is difficult. Most physicochemical characterizations have been accomplished using the virus particles present in stool specimens where sufficient numbers of virions can be obtained by ultracentrifugation/concentration.

Rotaviruses isolated from several animal species have shown a serological relationship with human rotaviruses (HRV). Antigenic crossings are demonstrated between HRV and rotaviruses isolated from calves, mice, and monkeys (table 20). In addition, the Nebraska calf diarrhea virus (NCDV) and the epidemic diarrhea of infant mice (EDIM) virus are both associated with gastroenteritis in infants of other species and in human infants, although simian virus (SA 11) and the related offal (O) agent isolated in South Africa are not known to be associated with a comparable syndrome.

Specimen Inoculation

Stool samples are the specimen of choice for visualization of the virus. Examination of duodenal mucosa at biopsy and of the intestinal contents, when available, are also suitable choices for obtaining virus. As yet tissue culture isolation methods are not available.

Virus Recognition and Assay

Direct detection by electron microscopy and immunoelectron microscopy. A 20% stool suspension, prepared in Hanks' BSS with a 0.5% bovine serum albumin free of antibody to human rotavirus (HRV), is centrifuged at 1000 × g for 30 minutes at 4°C to remove large debris and bacteria. The supernatant fluids can be stained with PTA and examined directly by EM. In certain instances, the supernatant fluids are sedimented at high-speed centrifugation (100,000 × g) for 1 hour. The pellet is resuspended in distilled water, and, after negative staining, examined by EM. The lowest limit of detection by this procedure is approximately 10^5 virus particles per gram of stool. If the number of virus

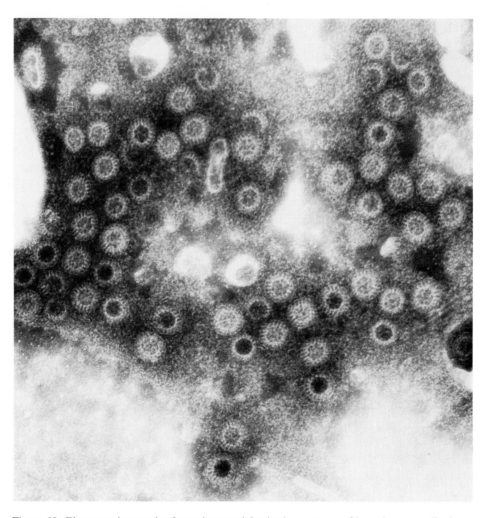

Figure 60. Electron micrograph of rotavirus particles in the presence of homologous antibody (IEM), negatively stained with PTA (100,800X).

Table 20. Antigenic Relationships among Rotaviruses Isolated from
Human and Nonhuman Sources

Animal Species (Virus Strain)	Source of Antigen	Levels of Antiserum Titers[a]				
		HRV	NCDV	EDIM	SA-11	O Agent
Human rotavirus (HRV)	stool filtrate	640	1024	1280	512	2048
Calf rotavirus (NCDV)	BEK cell cultures	1280	2048	1280	2048	8192
Mouse rotavirus (EDIM)	suckling mouse intestine	640	512	320	1024	4096
Simian rotavirus (SA-11)	GMK cell cultures	1280	2048	2560	2048	8192
Simian rotavirus (O agent)	GMK cell cultures	1280	2048	640	2048	4096

[a]Reciprocal dilutions of sera.
Source: Modified from A. Z. Kapikian et al., *Proc. Soc. Exp. Biol. and Med.* 152: 535, 1976.

particles in a stool specimen is very high, a water suspension of the stool can be examined directly without concentration procedures, in which case the specimen can be dried on a grid, washed, and negatively stained.

The immunoelectron microscopy techniques that have been developed are essential for identification of rotavirus. The partially purified, concentrated stool extract is mixed with appropriate dilutions of antiserum to rotavirus. After incubation (1 hour at room temperature), the mixture is applied to EM grids, negatively stained with PTA solution, and examined with an electron microscope. (For detailed procedure, see chapter 10). Figure 60 illustrates an aggregated rotavirus-antibody complex.

Scanning EM techniques have also been applied to cases of rotavirus infection. Examination of villi obtained from the small intestine during acute infection (approximately 48 hours after onset of the disease) reveals changes in appearance that are characteristic for rotavirus infection.

Detection of rotavirus in cell culture. Isolation of human rotavirus from clinical specimens is not as yet practical. Human embryonic kidney cell cultures showed limited growth for certain virus strains. Centrifugation of cell cultures inoculated with stool filtrates appears to increase sensitivity; 24 hours after incubation at 37°C, the infected cells can be detected by the IF technique using specific antiserum. Freshly trypsinized cells appear to be more sensitive to infection than established confluent monolayer cultures; apparently actively multiplying cells are more susceptible to rotavirus infection.

Detection of rotavirus by ELISA. Both direct and indirect ELISA methods have been adapted for the detection of rotavirus particles in stool samples. In the direct test, polyvinyl microtiter plates are precoated with rotavirus-specific antibody (capture antibody). After attachment of rotavirus particles to this specific antibody, a secondary rotavirus antibody, which has been conjugated with an enzyme, is added. Next is added a substrate, which is in turn converted by the enzyme to a visible color. The amount of color observed is directly proportional to the amount of rotavirus antigen present in the stool sample. The specific methodology is outlined and illustrated in detail in chapter 7.

Identification of Isolates

Immunoelectron microscopy (IEM). This was the method by which rotavirus infection in humans was first recognized. An 0.8 ml suspension of stool filtrate rich in rotavirus particles is mixed with 1:5 dilutions of acute or convalescent serum. The virus-serum mixture is incubated at room temperature for 1 hour, then overnight at 4°C to obtain the maximum amount of antibody-virus aggregates (see chapter 10).

Immunofluorescent test. As mentioned above, immune serum can be added to rotavirus-infected cell cultures and the infected cells can be detected by the indirect IF staining technique (see chapter 9).

Serodiagnosis

Rotavirus antibody can be detected and measured in microtiter plates by the ELISA. For details see chapter 7, in which rotavirus antigen is used as an example for ELISA methods.

SUPPLEMENTARY READING

Reovirus

Books and Review Papers

Joklik, W. Structure and function of the reovirus genome. *Microbiol. Rev.* 45: 483, 1981.
Rosen, L. Reoviruses. In *Diagnostic procedures for viral, rickettsial and chlamydial infections,* ed. E. H. Lennette and N. J. Schmidt, p. 577. 5th ed. Washington, D. C.: American Public Health Association, 1979.
Spendlove, R. S. Reoviridae: reoviruses. In *Virology and rickettsiology,* ed. G. D. Hsiung, and R. H. Green, vol. 1, pt. 1, p. 235. Handbook series in clinical laboratory science, Section H. West Palm Beach, Fla.: CRC Press, 1978.

Specific Articles

Gomatos, P. J., Tamm, I., Dales, S., and Franklin, R. M. Reovirus type 3: physical characteristics and interactions with L cells. *Virology* 17: 441, 1962.
Hsiung, G. D. Some distinctive biological characteristics of ECHO-10 virus. *Proc. Soc. Exp. Biol. Med.* 99: 387, 1958.
Rhim, J. S., Jordan, L. E., and Mayor, H. D. Cytochemical, fluorescent-antibody and

electron microscopic studies on the growth of reovirus (ECHO-10) in tissue cultures. *Virology* 17: 342, 1962.

Sabin, A. B. Reovirus: a new group of respiratory and enteric viruses formerly classified as ECHO type 10 is described. *Science* 130: 1387, 1959.

Weiner, H. L., and Field, B. N. Neutralization of reovirus: the gene responsible for the neutralization antigen. *J. Exp. Med.* 146: 1305, 1977.

Weiner, H. L., Ramig, R. F., Mustoe, T. A., and Fields, B. N. Identification of the gene coding for the hemagglutinin of reovirus. *Virology* 86: 581, 1978.

Zweerink, H. J., Morgan, E. M., and Skyler, J. S. Reovirus morphogenesis: characterization of subviral particles in infected cells. *Virology* 73: 442, 1976.

Rotavirus

Books and Review Papers

Kapikian, A. Z., Yolken, R. H., Greenberg, H. B., Wyatt, R. G., Kalica, A. R., Chanock, R. M., and Kim, H. W. Gastroenteritis viruses. In *Diagnostic procedures for viral, rickettsial and chlamydial Infections*, ed. E. H. Lennette and N. J. Schmidt, p. 927. 5th ed. Washington, D. C.: American Public Health Association, 1979.

Specific Articles

Bishop, R. F., Davidson, G. P., Holms, I. H., and Ruck, B. J. Virus particles in epithelial cells of duodenal mucosa from children with acute non-bacterial gastroenteritis. *Lancet* 2: 1281, 1973.

Flewett, T. H., Bryden, A. S., and Davies, H. Virus particles in gastroenteritis. *Lancet* 2: 1497, 1973.

Flewett, T. H., Diagnosis of enteritis virus. *Proc. Roy. Soc. Med.* (London) 69: 693, 1976.

Kapikian, A. Z., Cline, W. L., Kim, H. W., Kalica, A. R., Wyatt, R. G., VanKirk, D. H., Chanock, R. M., James, H. D., Jr., and Vaugh, A. C. Antigenic relationship among five reo-like (RVL) agents by complement fixation (CF) and development of a new substitute CF antigen for the human RVL agent of infantile gastroenteritis. *Proc. Soc. Exp. Biol. Med.* 152: 535, 1976.

Kapikian, A. Z., Kim, H. W., Wyatt, R. G., Rodriguez, W. G., Ross, S., Cline, W. L., Parrott, R. H., and Chanock, R. M. Reovirus like agent in stools' association with infantile diarrhea and development of serological tests. *Science* 185: 1049, 1974.

Moosai, R. B., Gardner, P. S., Almeida, J. D., and Greenaway, M. A. A simple immunofluorescent technique for the detection of human rotavirus. *J. Med. Virol.* 3: 189, 1979.

Roberton, D. M., Harrison, M., Hosking, C. S., Adams, L. C., and Bishop, R. F. Rapid diagnosis of rotavirus infection: comparison of electron microscopy and enzyme linked immunosorbent assay (ELISA). *Aust. Paediatr. J.* 15: 229, 1979.

Thouless, M. E., Bryden, A. S., Flewett, T. H., Wood, G. N., Bridger, J. C., Snodgrass, D. R., and Hersing, J. A. Serological relationships between rotaviruses from different species as studied by complement-fixation and neutralization. *Arch. Virol.* 53: 287, 1977.

Wood, G. N., Bridger, J. C., Jones, J. M., Flewett, T. H., Bryden, A. S., Davies, H. A., and White, G. G. G. Morphological and antigenic relationship between viruses (rotaviruses) from acute gastroenteritis of children, calves, piglets, mice and foals. *Inf. Imm.* 14: 804, 1976.

Yolken, R. H., Kim, H. W., Clem, T., Wyatt, R. G., Kalica, A. R., Chanock, R. M., and Kapikian, A. Z. Enzyme linked immunosorbent assay (ELISA) for detection of human reovirus-like agent of infantile gastroenteritis. *Lancet* 2: 263, 1977.

Yolken, R. H., and Stopa, P. J. Analysis of nonspecific reactions in enzyme-linked immunosorbent assay testing for human rotavirus. *J. Clin. Microbiol.* 10: 703, 1979.

Yolken, R. H., Wyatt, R. G., Zissis, G., et al. Epidemiology of human rotavirus types 1 and 2 as studied by enzyme-linked immunosorbent assay. *N. Eng. J. Med.* 299: 1156, 1978.

Zissis, G., and Lambert, J. P. Different serotypes of human rotavirus. *Lancet* 1: 38, 1978.

18. Rhabdoviridae

RABIES VIRUS AND VESICULAR STOMATITIS VIRUS

The rhabdoviridae includes the highly pathogenic rabies virus responsible for central nervous system (CNS) disease of man and animals as well as the relatively nonpathogenic vesicular stomatitis virus (VSV). The clinical symptoms associated with rabies virus include fever, convulsions, salivation, excitation, anxiety, difficulty in swallowing, and death. Tissues suspected of harboring rabies virus are sent to specifically designated centers for virus isolation and diagnosis. Animals suspected of having rabies virus infection (for example, bats trapped in houses), should be sent to state laboratories in order to maintain an epidemiologic surveillance of wildlife.

The rabies virion exhibits a bullet-shaped morphology with cylindrical particles, 60 × 180 nm. Each virion contains a single-stranded RNA nucleocapsid, which is surrounded by a lipid bilayer membrane with surface projections 6–8 nm in length. Rabies virions are observed in association with an intracytoplasmic filamentous matrix (figure 61). The virus is relatively stable in the presence of a stabilizing protein but is sensitive to ether treatment. In fixed tissue sections, the massed nucleocapsid material is recognized under light microscopy as intracytoplasmic inclusion bodies. The detection of Negri bodies in the Ammon's horn of the hippocampus and/or of rabies virus antigen in brain tissue by immunofluorescence are important diagnostic tools for rapid identification of rabies virus in animals suspected of being infected.

Vesicular stomatitis virus (VSV), morphologically similar to the rabies virus, grows well in cell culture. Since VSV is known to be relatively nonpathogenic to humans, it has been used commonly in the laboratory as a model for elucidating pathogenesis and morphogenesis of rhabdoviruses.

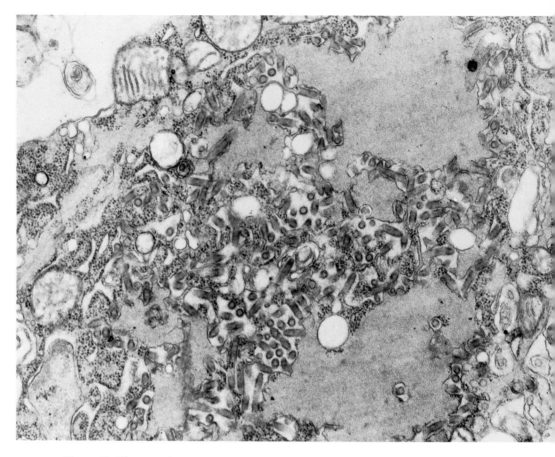

Figure 61. Electron micrograph of rabies virus particles in an infected mouse brain cell (25,000X) (F. A. Murphy, in *The natural history of rabies*, ed. G. M. Baer, New York: Academic Press, 1975, vol. 1, p. 33).

Specimen Inoculation

It is critically important to obtain a rapid diagnosis of rabies virus infection since immediate treatment with immune serum can result in survival without sequelae. There is usually a history of exposure to a bite of a dog, cat, wild animal, or bat; therefore, the selection of specimens is dictated by the assumption of exposure to a rabid animal. Saliva, throat swab, urine, and spinal fluid taken from suspected animals can be inoculated into 1- to 2-day-old mice.

Virus Isolation and Propagation

Virus isolation from wild animals for confirmation of diagnosis requires inoculation of suspected tissue in suspensions containing PBS, pH 7.2, with 0.75% bovine albumin into 1- to 2-day-old mice. The incubation period is from 5–12 days to as long as 3 weeks. Infected animals show paralysis and convulsions prior to death. Cell cultures are used in experimental studies but are not used for routine isolation procedures. Certain strains of rabies virus produce plaques in a strain of BHK-21/135 cells suspended in agarose.

Identification of Isolates

Direct examination of corneal epithelial cells for rabies antigen is a new test for the laboratory diagnosis of rabies either in humans or in animals. Slides with corneal impressions are air-dried, fixed in acetone, and stained with fluorescein-labeled rabies antiserum. However, a negative test does not rule out the possibility of rabies infection.

Rabies virus can be detected by direct microscopic examination of infected brains for Negri bodies and preferably for rabies virus antigen by direct immunofluorescent staining method. Identification of rabies virus in brain tissues can be made within hours using type-specific labeled rabies antibody. The neutralization test for virus identification depends on the use of known antiserum in order to reduce virus titer 100-fold or more as compared with known negative serum.

Examination of autopsy tissues by EM is another valuable means for direct visualization of the characteristic virus particles. Figure 61 illustrates a section of a rabies virus–infected mouse brain in which the bullet-shaped virus particles can be correlated with the intracellular inclusion of a neuron observed by light microscopy. Thin sections of VSV in cell culture and negatively stained virus particles (figure 62) illustrate a morphology similar to that seen in the rabies virus–infected brain cells.

Serodiagnosis

A neutralization test using newborn mice inoculated intracerebrally is commonly employed, although immunofluorescence tests are increasingly replacing other methods. The indirect immunofluorescent staining test using rabies virus–infected

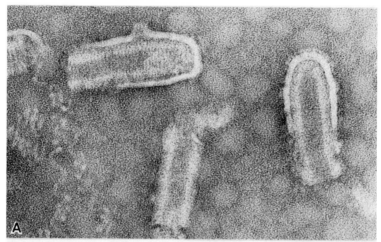

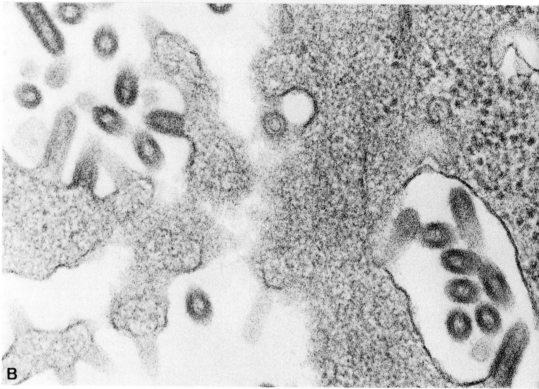

Figure 62. Electron micrographs of vesicular stomatitis virus (VSV).
A. Virus particles of bullet shape consisting of inner nucleocapsids and outer envelopes with projections, negatively stained with PTA (168,000X).
B. Thin section of a VSV-infected chick embryo cell showing virus particles budding into a cytoplasmic vacuole (100,800X).

180

cell cultures has been used for detecting antibody in human sera after rabies vaccination.

SUPPLEMENTARY READING

Books and Review Papers

Howatson, A. F. Vesicular stomatitis and related viruses. *Adv. Virus Res.* 16: 196, 1970.

Murphy, F. A. Morphology and morphogenesis. In *Natural history of rabies*, ed. G. M. Baer, vol. 1, p. 33. New York: Academic Press, 1975.

Shope, R. E. Rhabdoviridae: rabies and rabies-related viruses. In *Virology and rickettsiology,* ed. G. D. Hsiung and R. H. Green, vol. 1, pt. 1, p. 285. Handbook series in clinical laboratory science, Section H. West Palm Beach, Fla.: CRC Press, 1978.

Specific Articles

Cifuentes, E., Calderon, E., and Bijlenga, G. Rabies in a child diagnosed by a new intravitarn method: the cornea test. *J. Trop. Med. Hyg.* 74: 23, 1971.

Smith, J. S. ,Yager, P. A., and Baer, G. M. A rapid reproducible test for determining rabies neutralizing antibody. *Bull. W.H.O.* 48: 535, 1973.

Smith, W. B., Blenden, D. C., Fuh, T. H., and Hiler, L. Diagnosis of rabies by immunofluorescent staining of frozen sections of skin. *J. Am. Vet. Med. Assoc.* 161: 1495, 1972.

DNA VIRUSES

19. Adenoviridae

ADENOVIRUSES

The initial isolation of an adenovirus was made from a surgical specimen of human adenoid tissue, which, when grown in tissue culture, underwent spontaneous degeneration after prolonged incubation. Similar agents were subsequently recovered from patients with acute respiratory illness. It became apparent that adenoviruses are associated with a variety of clinical syndromes, including pharyngoconjunctival fever, acute febrile pharyngitis, and epidemic keratoconjunctivitis. More recently, new adenovirus types have been isolated from renal transplant recipients. To date 35 immunologically distinct types have been isolated from humans. Additional types have been recovered from chimpanzees, monkeys, dogs, cattle, chickens, and several other animal species, but each adenovirus type replicates best only in the tissues of the host from which the virus was isolated.

Electron microscopic examination of negatively stained preparations reveals that the adenoviruses are 70 to 80 nm in diameter (figures 63 and 64). Each virus particle consists of 252 capsomeres arranged in icosahedral symmetry: 240 hexons and 12 pentons, each of the latter attached with a fiber. In infected cells, adenovirus particles either singly (figure 63) or in groups (figure 64) are located in the nuclei. Chemical analysis indicates that the particles contain double-stranded DNA and are resistant to treatment with ether.

The majority of adenovirus types produce a characteristic cytopathic effect in tissue culture consisting of marked rounding and clumping, especially in serial lines such as Hep-2 or HeLa cells. Newly formed virus is usually cell-associated, and only a small percentage of virus is released into the culture field, even though marked CPE is observed. Virus multiplication is localized in the cell nucleus, and Feulgen-positive intranuclear inclusions are noted in stained preparations (color figures 5 and 6).

All adenoviruses, except those of the avian species, propagated in tissue cul-

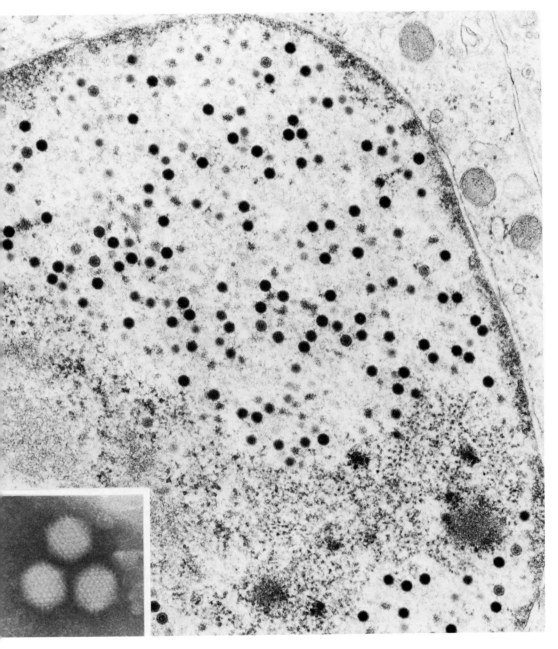

Figure 63. Electron micrograph of adenovirus type 2–infected human embryonic kidney (HEK) cell, showing virus particles scattered in the nucleus (38,400X) (modified from C. K. Y. Fong and G. D. Hsiung in *Virology and rickettsiology*, vol. 1, pt. 1, p. 88). Inset: Adenovirus particles stained with PTA (100,800X).

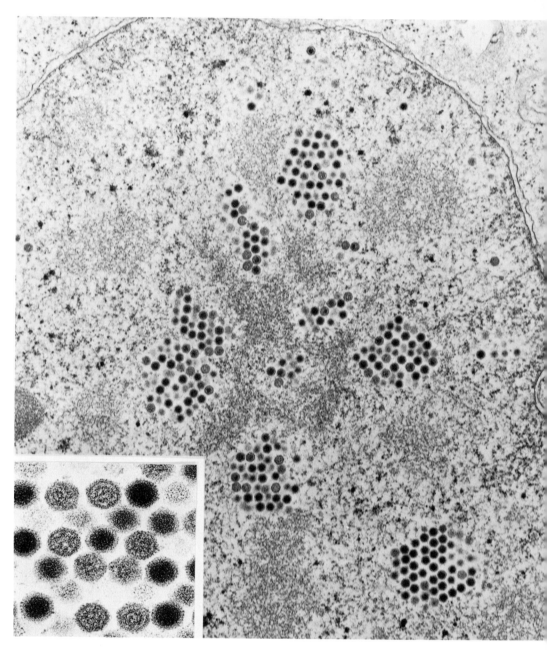

Figure 64. Electron micrograph of adenovirus type 7 in an infected HEK cell, showing virus aggregates in crystalline arrays in the nucleus (30,000X). Inset: Higher magnification of adenovirus particles in thin section (100,800X).

Table 21. Hemagglutination Properties of Human Adenoviruses

Group	Hemagglutination Monkey RBC	Rat RBC	Virus Types
I	+	−	3, 7, 11, 14, 16, 21, 34, 35
II	−	+	8, 9, 10, 13, 15, 17, 19, 20, 22–30, 32–33
III	−	P[a]	1, 2, 4, 5, 6, 12
IV	−	−	18, 31

[a]Partial hemagglutination or low hemagglutinin titers; this partial agglutination is rendered more evident or complete when the reaction is carried out in the presence of antibody to one of the heterologous types within the group.

Key: + = virus-induced change
 − = no change

ture produce a family-reactive soluble antigen, provided by the hexons, that can be detected by CF test. With a few exceptions, the adenoviruses isolated from humans agglutinate rhesus monkey or rat erythrocytes. Based upon these agglutinating properties, the human adenoviruses can be divided into four subgroups (table 21). Type 8, 9, 10, and 26 agglutinate human type-O erythrocytes as well.

Specimen Inoculation

Throat swabs, nasal swabs, eye swabs, and rectal swabs and/or stools are good sources for adenovirus isolation. These specimens can be inoculated directly into primary HEK cell cultures and passaged cell lines, including Hep-2, HeLa, KB, and A549, which are highly susceptible to human adenovirus infection. Cells from human amnion and kidney cells from certain monkey species are also susceptible to infection with some human adenovirus types.

Virus Isolation, Propagation, and Assay

Cytopathic effect in fluid cultures. The typical CPE of large grapelike clumps of degenerated cells produced by adenoviruses is usually recognized readily in HEK cultures (figures 65). Similar CPE occurs in Hep-2 cells 2 to 3 days after inoculation (figure 66). However, with the exception of laboratory-adapted human strains, onset of CPE is delayed in primary rhesus MK cell cultures (figure 67).

Since adenoviruses are cell-associated, both infected culture cells and fluids should be harvested. This is done by 2 or 3 cycles of freezing and thawing to release virus from infected cells. It is always good practice to subculture adenovirus-infected cells into the most highly sensitive cell cultures, i.e. human embryo kidney cells or A549 cells.

Cytopathology of infected cells. Adenoviruses produce typical intranuclear

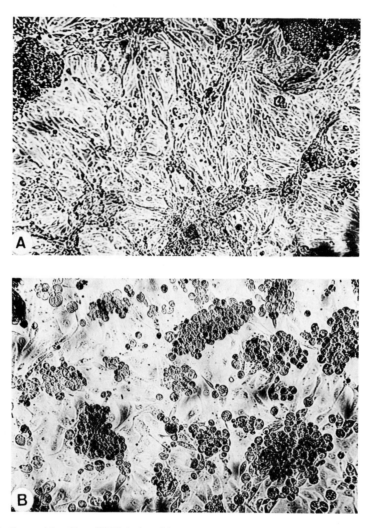

Figure 65. Cytopathic effect (CPE) induced by an adenovirus in HEK cell cultures (100X).
A. Uninfected HEK cultures.
B. CPE induced by adenovirus type 3.

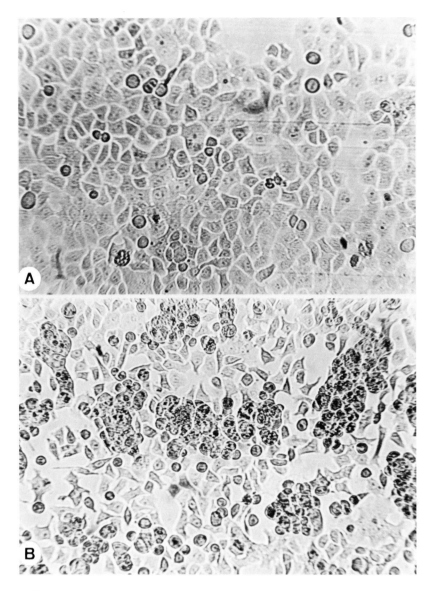

Figure 66. Cytopathic effect (CPE) induced by an adenovirus in Hep-2 cell cultures (100X).
    A. Uninfected Hep-2 culture.
    B. CPE induced by adenovirus type 3.

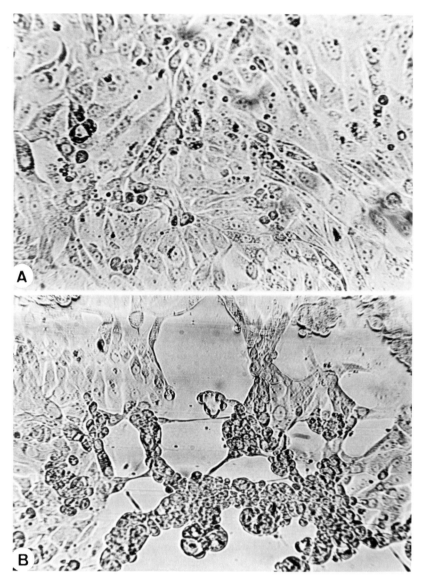

Figure 67. Cytopathic effect (CPE) induced by an adenovirus in RhMK cell cultures (100X).
  A. Uninfected RhMK culture.
  B. CPE induced by adenovirus type 3.

basophilic Feulgen-positive inclusions that are distinctly different from those produced by other viruses; they are illustrated in figures 68 and 69 and color figures 5 and 6. Inclusions can be recognized when infected cells are stained by hematoxylin-eosin or the Feulgen reaction method (see chapter 8). Inclusions produced by different adenovirus types show some degree of dissimilarity. One group, represented by adenovirus type 2, produces multiple well-defined eosinophilic intranuclear inclusions at an early stage of infection. Later these inclusions become Feulgen-positive basophilic granular clusters and are spaced throughout the nuclei (figure 68 and color figure 5). Another group, represented by adenovirus type 3, produces large basophilic inclusions that occupy the entire nucleus (figure 69). Since monkey kidney cells are not highly susceptible to human adenovirus, inclusions in MK cells are not distinct. Adenovirus types 1, 2, 5, and 6 produce similar changes, whereas the nuclear alterations induced by adenovirus types 3, 4, and 7 are almost identical with each other.

Identification of Isolates

Complement-fixation test. All known adenovirus types except those derived from the avian species have a family-reactive antigen. Hence, preliminary identification can be made by the CF test using a human adenovirus reference serum or antihexon serum. Standardization of the reagents used in the CF test, including Veronal buffer, hemolysin, and complement, is described in chapter 6. Human adenovirus reference sera are commonly used for preliminary identification of human adenovirus isolates.

Immunofluorescence or immunoperoxidase. All adenovirus-infected cells cross-react with antiserum to the common antigen, hexon, thus providing the basis for a relatively simple and rapid identification procedure utilizing indirect IP or IF techniques (see chapters 8 and 9). Figure 70 illustrates an example of cells infected with three adenovirus types reacting with a common reference serum in the IP method. However, these methods cannot be used for identifying adenovirus serotypes; the HI or neutralization tests, using type-specific antiserum, are necessary for type-specific identification.

Hemagglutination-inhibition test. All human adenoviruses except types 18 and 31 agglutinate either monkey or rat RBC. On the basis of their capacity to agglutinate RBC from different sources, adenoviruses can be divided into four subgroups (table 21). Subgroup I agglutinates monkey RBC; subgroups II and III agglutinate rat RBC. These biologic properties appear to be consistent with the subgrouping based on cytopathology in infected cells (see above). Subgroup III agglutinates rat RBC only partially; this partial agglutination is rendered more evident or complete when the reaction is carried out in the presence of antibody to the heterologous types within the group. For example, adenovirus type 12 agglutinates rat RBC only when antiserum to another member of group III (that is, adenovirus type 6 antiserum) is added to the system. The erythrocytes of individual rats or monkeys may or may not be agglutinable by the adenovirus types; therefore, RBC obtained from each animal should be tested

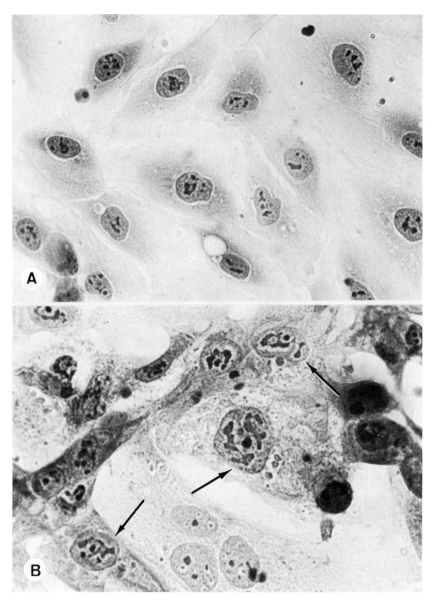

Figure 68. Basophilic intranuclear inclusions induced by adenovirus type 2 in HEK cell cultures (H&E, 400X).
A. Uninfected HEK cultures.
B. Basophilic inclusions (arrows) induced by adenovirus type 2.

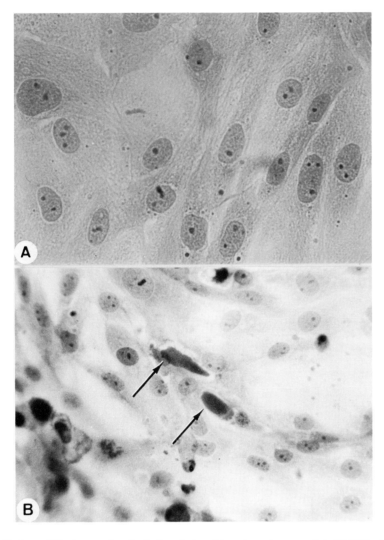

Figure 69. Basophilic intranuclear inclusions induced by adenovirus type 3 in RhMK cell cultures (H&E, 400X).
  A. Uninfected RhMK cultures.
  B. Basophilic intranuclear inclusions (arrows) induced by adenovirus type 3 in RhMK cells.

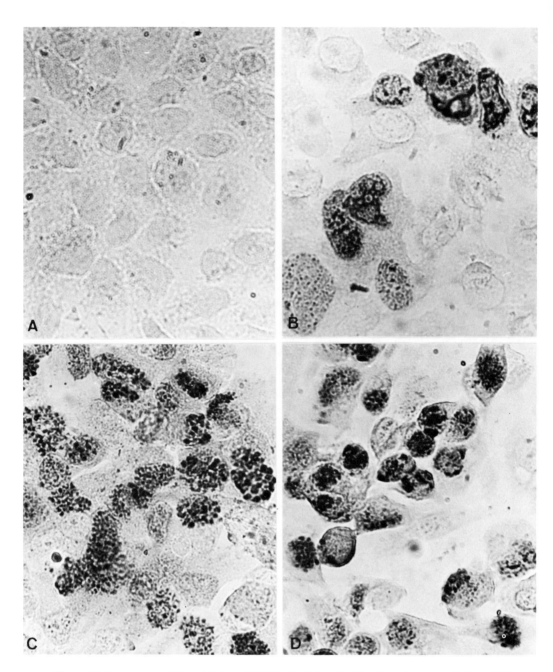

Figure 70. Immunoperoxidase staining of A549 cells infected with adenovirus types 2, 7, and 31, with an antiserum containing common antibody (400X) (courtesy of D. Brigati).
A. Uninfected A549 cell culture.
B. Intranuclear inclusion induced by adenovirus type 2.
C. Intranuclear inclusion induced by adenovirus type 7.
D. Intranuclear inclusion induced by adenovirus type 31.

before they are used for HA or HI. The concentrations of monkey or rat RBC and the suitable diluents are listed in table 4 on page 36. Thus, the HI test can be used to identify most of the adenovirus types using either rat or monkey RBC and type-specific antiserum.

Neutralization test in tissue culture. No hemagglutinins can be demonstrated for adenovirus types 18 and 31. Thus these two types, as well as those that give only partial hemagglutination, are commonly identified by neutralization tests using type-specific antiserum in a cell culture system. A challenge dose of 30 to 50 $TCID_{50}$ is often used. The inhibition of virus-induced CPE is far more sensitive than the HI test for the identification of these adenovirus types.

Electron microscopy. Electron microscopy has been used widely for studying the sequential changes associated with adenovirus replication. Occasionally, certain adenoviruses that cannot be cultivated in cell culture are recognized in negatively stained preparations of stool specimens. Electron microscopic examination of thin sections prepared from adenovirus-infected cells frequently reveals characteristic virus particles in crystalline arrays in the nuclei of infected cells. Although adenoviruses can be identified by many other methods, as mentioned above, electron microscopy is and will be a very useful tool in the recognition of viruses in this group.

Serodiagnosis

Rise in antibody titers to the adenovirus group antigen or hexon, regardless of specific immunotype, by the CF test with paired sera is an indication of a recent adenovirus infection. Type-specific rises are detected by means of HI or neutralization tests. As with other serologic tests, only a 4-fold or greater rise is of diagnostic significance.

Oncogenic Properties of Adenoviruses

Initially, adenovirus types 12, 18, and 31 were found capable of producing tumors in newborn hamsters; subsequently, additional types, including adenovirus types 3, 7, 11, 14, 16, and 21, showed similar effect. Since then these strains, especially adenovirus type 12, have been used extensively for studies of viral oncogenic properties in cultured cells as well as in experimental animals.

SUPPLEMENTARY READING

Books and Review Papers

Ginsberg, H. S. Adenoviruses. In *Virology*, ed. R. Dubecco and H. S. Ginsberg, p. 1047. 3rd ed. Harperstown, Md.: Harper and Row, Inc., 1980.

Ledinko, N. Adenoviridae. In *Virology and rickettsiology*, ed. G. D. Hsiung and R. H. Green, vol. 1, pt. 2, p. 43. Handbook series in clinical laboratory science, Section H. West Palm Beach, Fla.: CRC Press, 1978.

Specific Articles

Hierholzer, J. C., Atuk, N. O., and Gwaltney, J. M. New human adenovirus isolated from renal transplant recipient, description and characterization of candidate adenovirus type 34. *J. Clin. Microbiol.* 1:366–76, 1975.

Huebner, R. J., Rowe, W. P., and Lane, W. T. Oncogenic effects in hamsters of human adenovirus types 12 and 18. *Proc. Nat. Acad. Sci.* (Wash.) 48: 2051, 1962.

Myerowitz, R. L., Stalker, H., Oxman, M. N., Levin, N. J., Moore, M., Leith, J. D., Gantz, N. M., and Pellegrini, J. Fatal disseminated adenovirus infection in a renal transplant recipient. *Am. J. Med.* 57: 591–97, 1975.

Rowe, W. P., Heubner, R. J., Gilmore, L. K., Parrott, R. H., and Ward, T. C. Isolation of a cytopathogenic agent from human adenoids undergoing spontaneous degeneration in tissue culture. *Proc. Soc. Exp. Biol. Med.* 84: 570, 1953.

Sullivan, E. F., and Rosenbaum, M. J. Isolation and identification of adenoviruses in microplates. *Appl. Microbiol.* 22: 802, 1971.

Trentin, J. J., Yabe, Y., and Taylor, G. The quest for human cancer viruses. *Science* 137: 835, 1962.

Wang, S. S., and Feldman, H. A. Pharyngeal isolations of adenovirus 31 from a family population. *Am. J. Epidemiol.* 104: 272, 1976.

20. Herpesviridae

All herpesviruses are morphologically similar but biologically they are distinctly different from one another. Based upon their biologic and serologic properties, five distinct herpesviruses infecting humans (table 22) have been characterized. These are herpes simplex virus (HSV) types 1 and 2, varicella-zoster virus (VZV), cytomegalovirus (CMV), and Epstein-Barr virus (EBV). Occasionally a herpesvirus of monkeys (herpesvirus simiae, the B virus) has been known to infect humans.

Herpesviruses have been isolated from many lower animal species, including rabbits, guinea pigs, mice, rats, squirrels, and even frogs. Infection with herpesviruses in man may take several diverse forms and often is inapparent. After a primary infection, either clinical or subclinical, an individual may become a carrier of latent virus even though specific neutralizing antibody may be present. The person with herpes simplex is commonly subject to recurrent vesicular eruptions. The virus can be readily isolated from these "fever blisters" (or "cold sores") or from vesicle fluids.

Mature herpesvirus particles range from 150 to 200 nm and contain a central DNA core. Each virus particle consists of 162 capsomeres surrounded by a double membrane–bound lipoprotein envelope (figure 71). The virus is extremely labile and readily inactivated by a lipid solvent such as diethyl ether. In addition, multiplication of the virus can be easily inhibited by a DNA inhibitor, for example 5-bromo-2′-deoxyuridine, a method commonly used to determine viral nucleic acid type. Virus multiplication occurs in the nucleus. Intranuclear Cowdry type A inclusions, each surrounded by a halo, are often seen in infected cells.

Table 22. Host Cell Spectrum and Pathogenicity of Human Herpesviruses

Virus Type	Sources of Specimen	Cytopathic Effect in Cell Culture Systems					Pathogenicity in	
		MK	HDF	Hep-2	RK	CE	Newborn Mice	Embryonated Eggs
Herpes simplex virus type 1 (HSV-1)	vesicle fluid or throat swab	+/−	+	+	+ +	−	+	+ (pinpoint pocks)
Herpes simplex virus type 2 (HSV-2)	vesicle fluid or genital lesions	+/−	+	+	+ +	+	+	+ (large pocks)
Varicella-zoster virus (VZV)	lesion swab, vesicle fluid	−	+ +	−	−	−	−	−
Cytomega-lovirus (CMV)	urine, saliva, milk, and cervical swab	−	+ +	−	−	−	−	−
Epstein-Barr virus (EBV)	blood, leukocytes,[a] throat swab[b]	−	−	−	−	−	−	−

[a]Cultivation of leukocytes.
[b]Virus in throat swab can be used for transforming leukocytes.

Key: + = virus-induced change
       − = no change

HERPES SIMPLEX VIRUS

Specimen Inoculation

Vesicular fluids, throat swabs, and genital lesions are sources for virus isolation. Best results are obtained when specimens are freshly collected and inoculated immediately into cell cultures. Both herpes simplex virus types 1 and 2 have a wide host spectrum, thus the specimens can be inoculated into a variety of tissue culture systems. Both primary cell cultures and cell lines derived from human and nonhuman origin are susceptible to HSV infection. Rapid growth of HSV in rabbit kidney cells and other cells of nonprimate origin, including guinea pig embryo cells, is an *important* characteristic since most human viruses do not generally replicate in nonprimate cell types. Most of the herpes simplex virus strains isolated from oral herpetic lesions are type 1; most of those isolated from genital lesions are type 2.

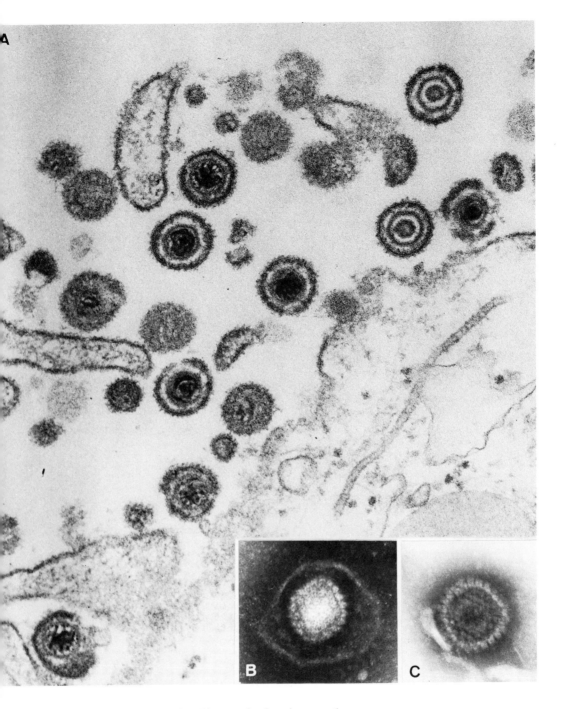

Figure 71. Electron micrographs of herpes simplex virus type 1.
    A. Thin section of an infected rabbit kidney cell culture showing many extracellular
       enveloped virus particles (100,800X).
    B. Enveloped herpesvirus particle stained with PTA (165,000X).
    C. Naked nucleocapsid stained with PTA (168,000X).

Virus Isolation, Propagation, and Assay

Cytopathic effect in fluid cultures. Herpes simplex virus induces rapid cellular degeneration in many cell types including those of nonprimate origins (for example, RK cells) as well as cells of human origin including HEK, HEF, HeLa, and Hep-2. Clusters of degenerated cells can be readily observed in infected RK and Hep-2 cell cultures (figure 72). However, CPE usually is not distinct in rhesus monkey kidney cells although green monkey kidney cells are sensitive. Since extensive CPE occurs rapidly in RK cells, usually within 24 hours when virus concentrations are high, RK cells are the most suitable system for the isolation and recognition of HSV.

Cytopathology in stained preparations. In hematoxylin-eosin-stained preparations, intranuclear inclusions are basophilic in nature (figure 73) and Feulgen-positive. As the infection progresses, the virus particles move from the nucleus into the cytoplasm and the inclusions are converted into an eosinophilic, Feulgen-negative mass. Thus, when eosinophilic inclusions are observed, there are fewer identifiable virus particles present.

Mouse pathogenicity. Although newborn mice are not commonly used for isolation of herpes simplex virus in the laboratory, it should be noted that after intracerebral or intraperitoneal inoculation, they develop a characteristic encephalitis. Cowdry type A inclusions are usually found in the hematoxylin-eosin-stained sections of infected mouse brain tissue.

Plaque formation. Plaque formation has been used for assaying HSV either in bottle cultures under agar overlay medium or in plastic plate cultures under methylcellulose overlay (see chapter 4). Distinct plaques appear 2–3 days after inoculation (figure 74) and are easily enumerated.

Identification of Isolates

Differentiation of HSV and other human herpesviruses. The typical CPE induced by HSV in cell culture, the wide host-infectivity range, and the relatively rapid growth rate permit the prompt recognition of HSV infection in cell culture.

Indirect immunofluorescent staining technique using specific antiserum is the most useful and rapid method for distinguishing herpes simplex virus from varicella-zoster virus and cytomegalovirus. However, this method cannot be used for typing HSV-1 and HSV-2 without further manipulation.

Neutralization with specific herpes simplex virus antiserum in cell culture, either by inhibition of CPE or plaque reduction, can be performed for final identification of HSV. However, both neutralization and IF tests cannot be easily applied for differentiating between HSV-1 and HSV-2 since antigenic crossing between the two is extensive (figure 7, bottom panel).

Differentiation of herpes simplex virus types 1 and 2. Advantage has been taken of the fact that HSV-2 has the ability to produce plaques in CE cells whereas HSV-1 does not (figure 74). This biologic property of cell culture selectivity offers a great advantage for differentiating these two virus types,

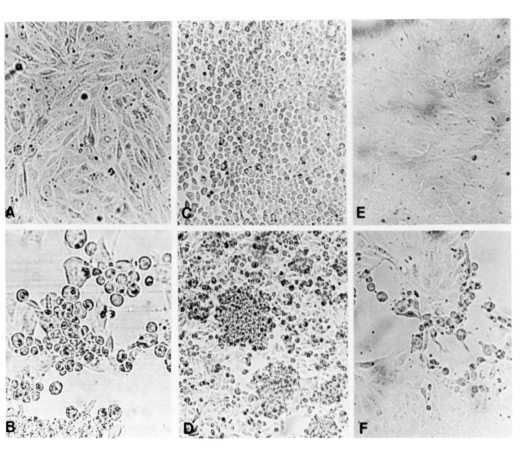

Figure 72. Cytopathic effect (CPE) induced by herpes simplex virus type 1 in different cell
cultures (100X).
A. Uninfected RK cell culture.
B. CPE induced by HSV-1 in RK cells, 1 day after inoculation.
C. Uninfected Hep-2 cell culture.
D. CPE induced by HSV-1 in Hep-2 cells, 2 days after inoculation.
E. Uninfected RhMK cell culture.
F. CPE induced by HSV-1 RhMK cells, 4 days after inoculation.

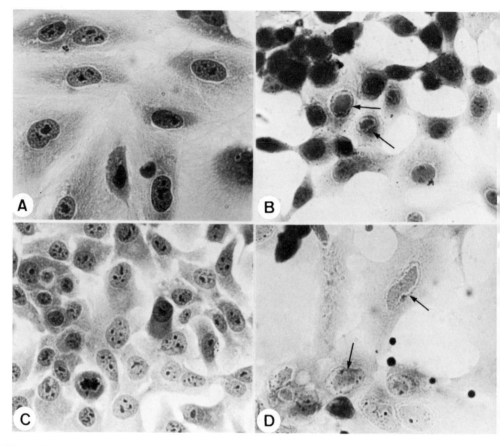

Figure 73. Intranuclear inclusions induced by herpes simplex virus in HEK and Hep-2 cell
cultures, 24 hours after infection (H&E, 400X).
A. Uninfected HEK culture.
B. Basophilic and eosinophilic inclusions (arrows) induced by herpes simplex virus in
HEK cells.
C. Uninfected Hep-2 culture.
D. Basophilic and eosinophilic inclusions (arrows) induced by herpes simplex virus in
Hep-2 cells.

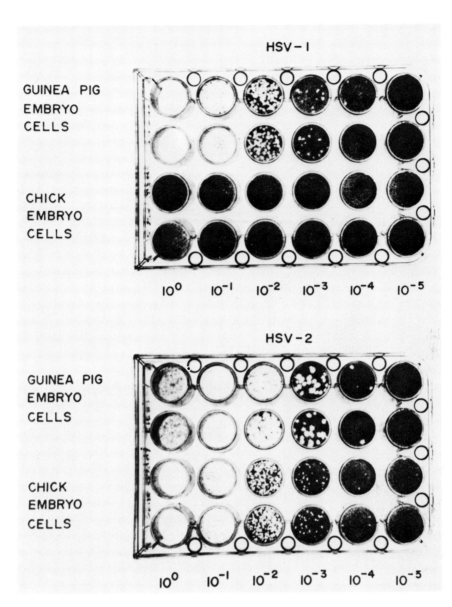

Figure 74. Typing of HSV-1 and HSV-2 by cell culture selection. Top: HSV-1 induces plaques in GPE cells but not in CE cells. Bottom: HSV-2 induces plaques in both GPE and CE cell cultures (Original photos, courtesy of M. J. August).

especially when cross-reactivity is encountered in the serologic tests, for example using IF test. Similarly, chorioallantoic membranes (CAM) can also be used for differentiation of the two types: HSV-1 produces pinpoint minute pocks on the CAM of embryonated eggs, whereas HSV-2 produces large clear pocks.

Electron microscopy. Direct visualization of herpesvirus particles in thin sections of infected cells or in negatively stained preparations provides an important tool for rapid diagnosis, which is especially important in cases of herpes encephalitis where effective chemotherapeutic measures can be applied. Distinct nucleocapsids, either in groups or scattered, are easily recognizable in the infected cells obtained from brain biopsy (figure 75) or in cultured cells (figures 76 and 77). In addition, HSV-2 often induces fibers (figure 77B), which appear to be a distinct morphologic characteristic that is lacking in HSV-1 cells.

Serodiagnosis

The complement-fixation test has been commonly used for demonstration of antibody rise to primary herpes simplex virus infection. Patients with recurrent disease have a high initial HSV antibody titer; thus they do not show a significant antibody rise and the test has a limited diagnostic value.

VARICELLA-ZOSTER VIRUS AND CYTOMEGALOVIRUS

Specimen Inoculation

Vesicle fluid and lesion swabs are good sources for VZV isolation, whereas urine, saliva and genital secretions often contain large numbers of CMV particles. Since these viruses are extremely labile, it is best to inoculate specimens at bedside. Human fibroblast cells, such as WI-38, and human fetal diploid cell lines are sensitive to both human CMV and VZV infection. Serial propagation of CMV and more particularly of VZV is accomplished best by transferring intact infected cells. Freshly collected urine samples are used for CMV isolation attempts, although virus particles can be observed in stored urine samples under electron microscopic examination.

Virus Isolation, Propagation, and Assay

In contrast to HSV, human CMV and VZV do not ordinarily induce CPE in cells other than those of human origin, nor do these two viruses cause disease in experimental animals, including newborn mice and chick embryos.

Cytopathic effect in fluid culture. Varicella-zoster virus isolation requires 3–7 days of cultivation. VZV grows slowly in human fibroblasts with focal CPE, but not in RK cells (figure 78). This is in contrast to HSV, which induces extensive CPE in both HDF and RK cells. Subculture of VZV to fresh cultures requires transfer of intact infected cells.

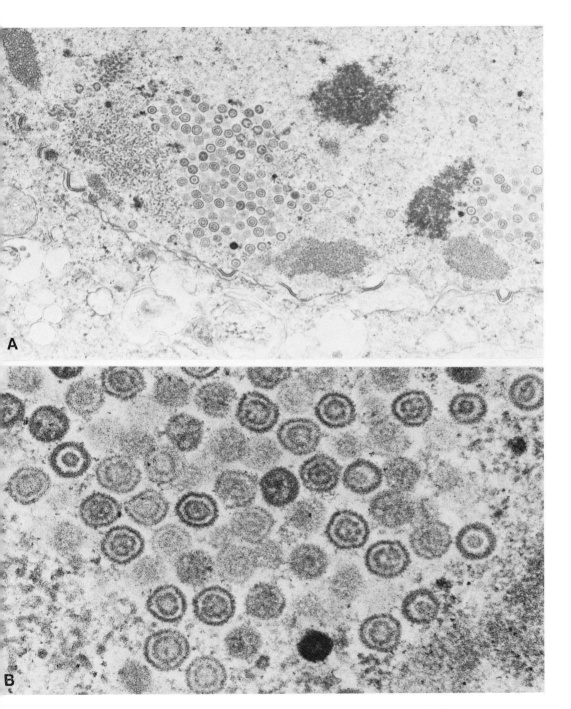

Figure 75. Electron micrograph of HSV-1 in an infected neuron from a human brain biopsy
(courtesy of M. J. August).
   A. Aggregates of nucleocapsids in the nucleus (24,000X).
   B. Higher magnification of nucleocapsids in (A) (100,800X) (modified from C. K. Y.
      Fong and G. D. Hsiung, in *Virology and rickettsiology*, vol. 1, pt. 1, p. 94).

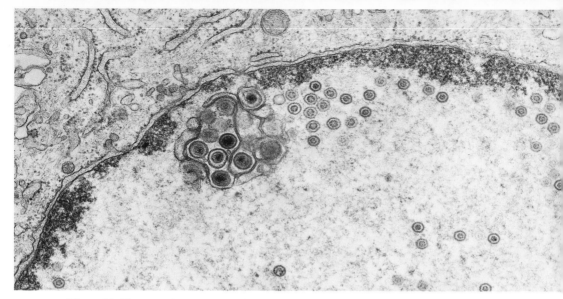

Figure 76. Electron micrograph of HSV-1 in an infected rabbit kidney cell, showing viral nucleocapsids and enveloped virus particles in the nucleus (30,000X).

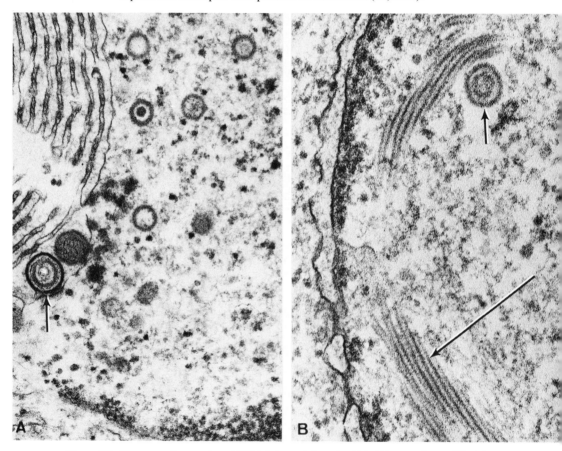

Figure 77. Electron micrographs of HSV-2 in an infected rabbit kidney cell (modified from
C. K. Y. Fong and G. D. Hsiung, in *Virology and rickettsiology*, vol. 1, pt. 1, p. 93).
  A. Portion of a nucleus containing viral nucleocapsids, enveloped virus particles
     (arrow), and membrane duplication (64,800X).
  B. Portion of a nucleus showing filamentous structures (long arrow) induced by
     HSV-2 (short arrow) (100,800X).

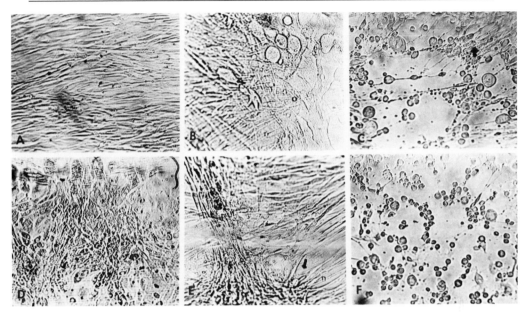

Figure 78. Cytopathic effect (CPE) induced by VZV and HSV in HDF and RK cells (100X)
(modified from M. L. Landry and G. D. Hsiung, *Conn. Med.* 45: 418, 1981).
A. Uninfected HDF (WI-38) cells.
B. Focal CPE induced by VZV in HDF cells.
C. Extensive CPE induced by HSV-1 in HDF cells.
D. Uninfected RK cells.
E. Absence of CPE in RK cells inoculated with VZV.
F. Extensive CPE induced by HSV-1 in RK cells.

Similarly, cytomegalovirus also induces cellular changes in human fibroblast cell culture but not in RK cells. Focal areas of rounded, enlarged cells (figure 79) occur 7 to 10 days after inoculation of HDF cells, although sometimes after 2 to 3 weeks of incubation. In both instances it is always advisable to allow specimens to adsorb onto the monolayer cultures for 2 to 4 hours after inoculation before fresh medium is added.

Cytopathology in stained preparations. Both VZV and CMV induce intranuclear inclusions in infected cells. The Cowdry type A nuclear inclusions typical of CMV infection (figure 80) are eosinophilic (color figure 7) in hematoxylin-eosin-stained preparations.

Identification of Isolates

Presumptive diagnosis of cytomegalovirus infection in children is often made from the observation of characteristic cytomegalic cells in the urine sediment. In most laboratories, identification of cytomegalovirus isolates is based on their pathogenic cytopathology, slow growth rate, and narrow host range in cell culture. VZV is commonly isolated from vesicle fluids. It also possesses a narrow host range which easily separates VZV from HSV.

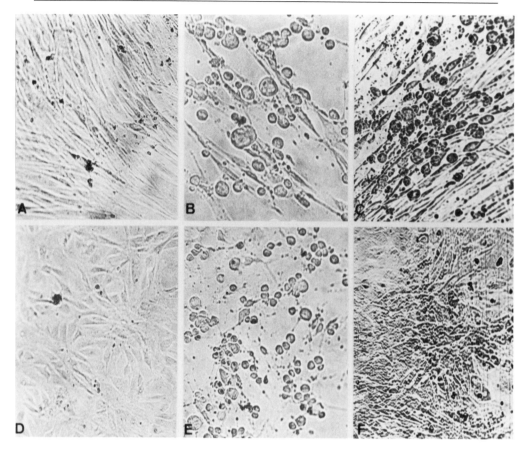

Figure 79. Cytopathic effect (CPE) induced by CMV and HSV in HDF and RK cells (100X).
    A. Uninfected HDF cell.
    B. CPE induced by HSV-1 in HDF cells.
    C. CPE induced by CMV in HDF cells.
    D. Uninfected RK cells.
    E. Extensive CPE induced by HSV-1 in RK cells.
    F. Absence of CPE in RK cells inoculated with CMV.

Virus isolates also can be identified by indirect IF staining technique on virus-infected cells or by CF test using type-specific antiserum to CMV or VZV.

Electron microscopy. The use of negative staining and EM examination of urine sediment for detecting CMV in congenitally infected infants or in immunocompromised patients has been very helpful. The distinct herpesvirus morphology is easily identified (figure 81). Similarly, herpesvirus particles are also easily found in lesion fluids obtained from patients with chicken pox (figure 81). However, a somewhat different ultrastructure is often seen in VZV- and CMV-infected cells (figures 82 and 83). For example, particles containing dense bodies are found only in CMV-infected cells (figure 82), whereas the virus particles seen in VZV-infected cells are often distorted (figure 83).

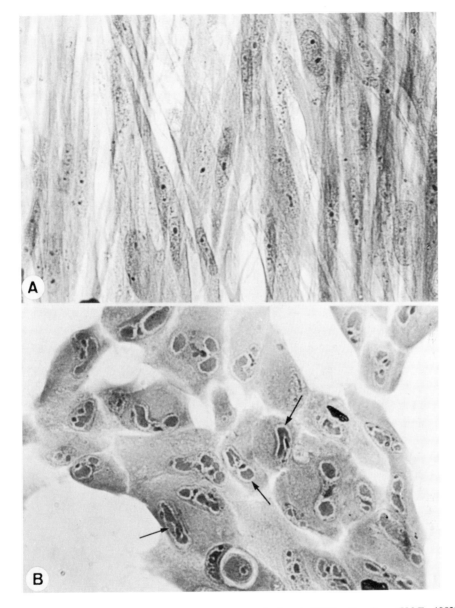

Figure 80. Intranuclear inclusions by human cytomegalovirus in HDF cell culture (H&E, 400X).
    A. Uninfected HDF.
    B. Eosinophilic intranuclear inclusions (arrows) in HDF cells.

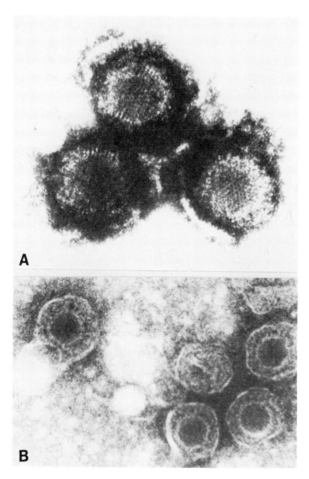

Figure 81. Negative staining of herpesvirus particles in clinical specimens.
        A. Cytomegalovirus particles seen in a urine sample stained with PTA (150,000X)
           (F. K. Lee, et al., *New Engl. J. Med.* 299: 1266, 1978).
        B. Varicella-zoster virus particles seen in vesicular lesions, stained with PTA
           (65,000X) (F. W. Doane and N. Anderson, in *Comparative diagnosis of viral*
           diseases, ed. E. Kurstak and C. Kurstak, New York: Academic Press, 1977,
           vol. 2, p. 512).

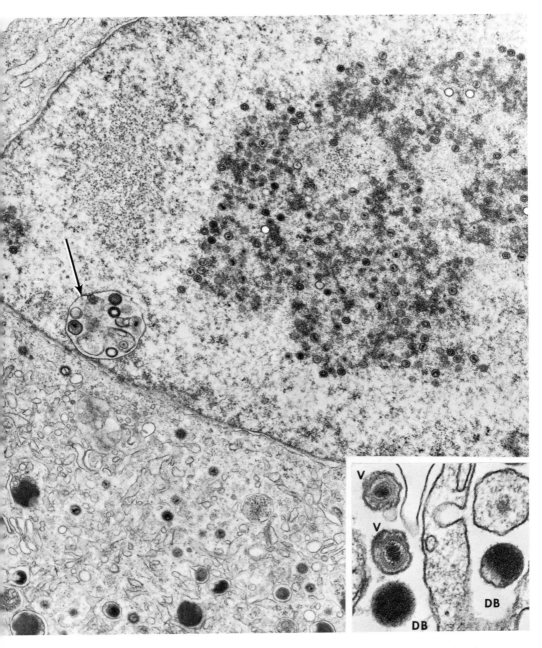

Figure 82. Electron micrograph of a human cytomegalovirus–infected HDF cell, showing intranuclear inclusion containing scattered viral nucleocapsids. A few enveloped virus
particles inside a vacuole are indicated by an arrow (19,680X). Inset: Enveloped
mature virus particles (V) and dense bodies (DB) (64,800X).

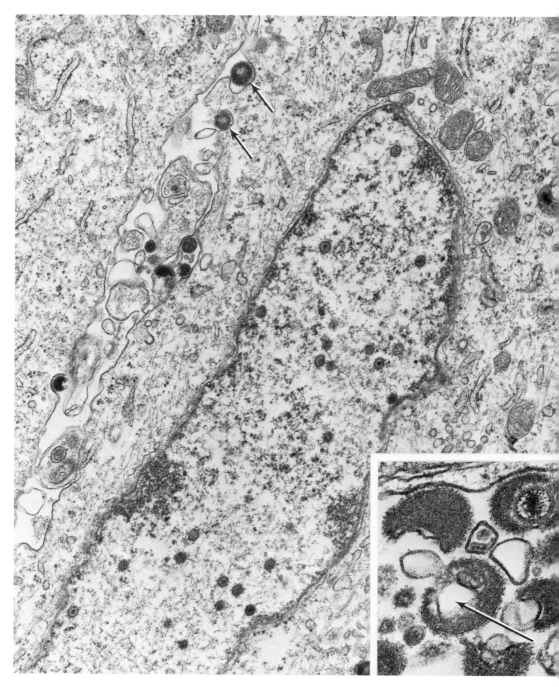

Figure 83. Electron micrograph of varicella-zoster virus (VZV) in an infected HDF cell. Many
nucleocapsids are scattered in the nucleus; a few enveloped virus particles are seen at
the extracellular space (arrows) (30,000X). Inset: Higher magnification of enveloped
extracellular virus particles; virus particles are devoid of nucleocapsids (arrow),
characteristic for VZV (100,800X).

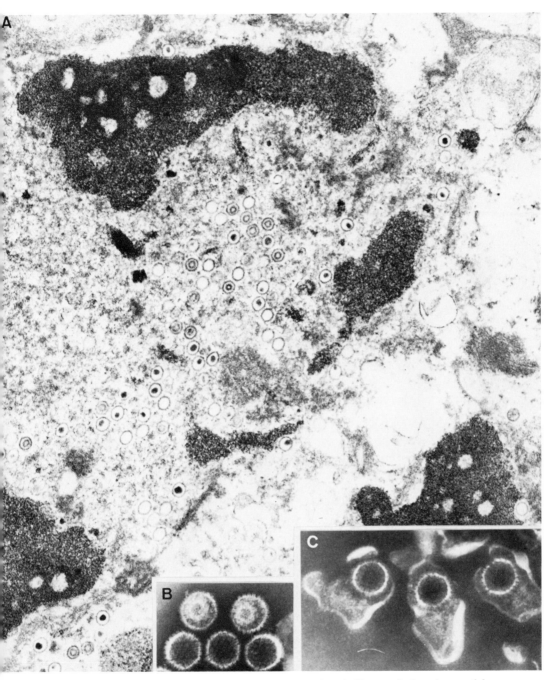

Figure 84. Electron micrographs of EBV and EBV-infected lymphoblast producing virus particles
(modified from G. Miller, *J. Inf. Dis*. 130: 187, 1974).
   A. Thin section of an EBV producer cell, showing many viral nucleocapsids in the
      nucleus at various stages of development (43,560X).
   B. Purified EBV nucleocapsids stained with PTA (101,000X).
   C. Enveloped EBV particles stained with PTA (101,000X).

Table 23. EBV-Related Antigen-Antibody System

Antigen Tested	Lymphoblast Line	Antibody Determination	
		Method Used	Positive Serum from
Viral capsid antigen (VCA)	smears with virus-producing cells	indirect IF	EBV carriers
Cell membrane antigen (MA), early and late	suspension containing abortively infected nonproducer cells, not fixed	inhibition of direct IF	most EBV carriers
Early antigen (EA), diffused and restricted	smears with abortively EBV superinfected nonproducer cells	inhibition of indirect IF, direct IF	infectious mononucleosis and nasopharyngeal carcinoma patients Burkitt's lymphoma patients
EBV nuclear antigen (EBNA)	smears of non-producer cells	anti-com-plement IF	EBV carriers
Soluble antigen	extract from nonproducer cells	CF	EBV carriers
Enveloped virus particles	producer virus culture fluid concentrate	NT	all EBV carriers

Source: Modified from W. Henle, G. Henle, and C. A. Horwitz, in *Diagnostic procedures for viral, rickett-sial and chlamydial infection*, ed. E. H. Lennette and N. J. Schmidt, p. 446 (1979).

Serodiagnosis

Since virus isolation is often slow and difficult, serologic tests have been most helpful in the confirmation of diagnosis when acute and convalescent serum samples are available.

Complement-fixation test is the most common method for assaying antibody rise to infection with CMV or VZV. Although it is not as sensitive as the immunofluorescent assay or neutralization test, it is the most inexpensive and convenient method for serodiagnosis. CF antigens for CMV and VZV are available commercially. More recently ELISA has been applied to the detection of antibody to CMV or VZV in patients suspected of being infected with these viruses.

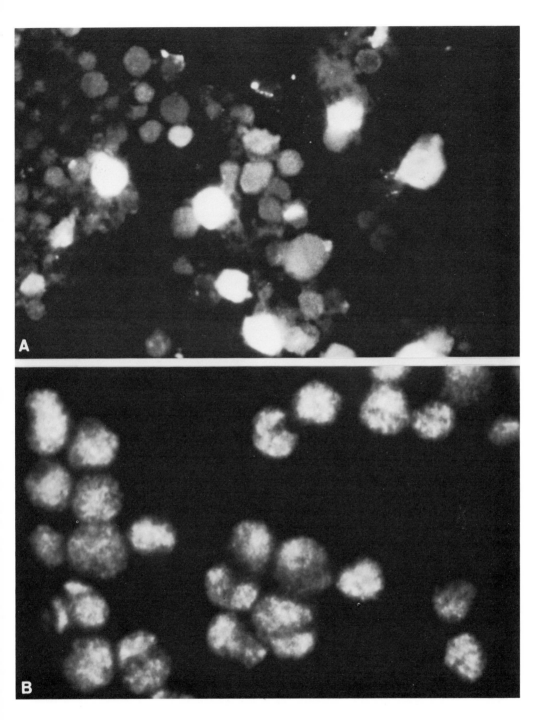

Figure 85. Immunofluorescent staining of EBV producer cells with patient serum (400X) (courtesy of W. Henle, University of Pennsylvania).
   A. Positive serum showing antibody to VCA in EB$_3$ cells.
   B. Positive serum showing antibody to EBNA.

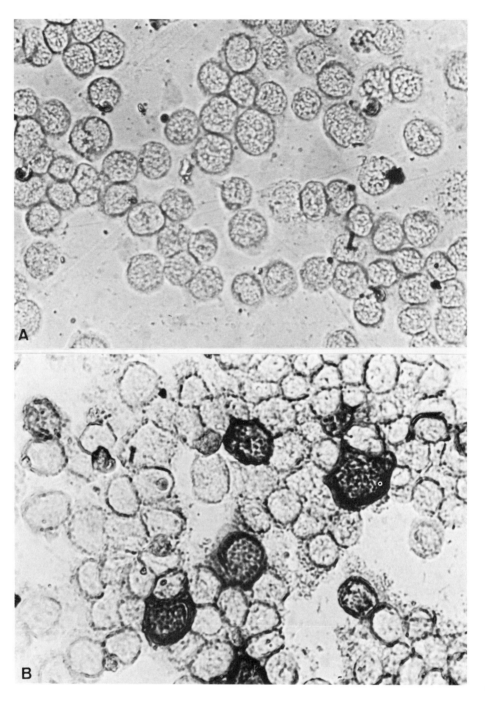

Figure 86. Immunoperoxidase staining of B95-8 cells with patient serum (400X).
    A. Patient serum without antibody.
    B. Serum from patient with nasopharyngeal carcinoma showing positively stained
       B95-8 cells (original slide obtained from G.-Y. Wu of Hunan Medical College,
       Changsha, Hunan, P.R.C.).

EPSTEIN-BARR VIRUS

Epstein-Barr virus (EBV) is another herpesvirus that infects man. Although virus particles have been observed in cultured cells derived from Burkitt's lymphoma tissue and from leukocytes of peripheral blood of infectious mononucleosis patients (figure 84), the isolation of cell-free transmissible viral agents is not commonly attempted.

Demonstration of EB herpesvirus infection requires cultivation of lymphocytes taken from patients or ability to transform cord blood leukocytes. Therefore, serologic tests are the most useful method for laboratory diagnosis of EBV infection.

Serodiagnosis

Routinely, the heterophil-antibody technique has been applied for the diagnosis of infectious mononucleosis. In recent years the immunofluorescent staining technique has been applied to detect the various EBV-related antigens (table 23). The differentiation of virus-specific antigens and the development of the corresponding antibodies are indications of the status of the EBV infection. Thus, a single serum can be used for detection of the various specific antibodies against the various cells containing each specific antigenic property. The IF test has been used for detection of antibodies to the various antigenic components of EBV, for example, viral capsid antigen (VCA) or EBV nuclear antigen (EBNA) (figure 85). More recently, the IP test has been applied for detecting IgM and IgG antibody to EBV-capsid antigen (figure 86).

SUPPLEMENTARY READING

Herpes Simplex Virus

Books and Review Papers

Baringer, J. Herpes simplex virus infection of nerve tissue in animals and man. *Prog. Med. Virol.* 20:1, 1975.

Nahmias, A. J., Dowdle, W. R., and Schinazi, R. F., eds. *The human herpesviruses.* New York: Elsevier, 1981.

Nahmias, A. J., and Roizman, B. Infection with herpes simplex viruses 1 and 2. *N. Eng. J. Med.* 286: 667, 719 and 781, 1973.

Specific Articles

Buchman, T. G., Roizman, B., Adams, G., and Stover, B. H. Restriction endonuclease fingerprinting of herpes simplex virus DNA: a novel epidemiology tool applied to a nosocomial outbreak. *J. Infect. Dis.* 138: 488, 1978.

Landry, M. L., Mayo, D. R., and Hsiung, G. D. Comparison of guinea pig embryo cells, rabbit kidney cells and human embryonic lung fibroblast cell strains for the isolation of herpes simplex virus. *J. Clin. Micro.* 15: 842, 1982.

Moseley, R. C., Corey, L., Banjamin, D., Winter, C., and Remington, M. L. Comparison of viral isolation, direct immunofluorescence, and indirect immunoperoxidase techniques for detection of genital herpes simplex virus infection. *J. Clin. Micro.* 13: 913, 1981.

Nahmias, A., DelBuono, I., Pipkin, J., Hutton, K., and Wickliffe, C. Rapid identification and typing of herpes simplex virus types 1 and 2 by a direct immunofluorescence technique. *Appl. Micro.* 22: 455, 1971.

Nordlund, J. J., Anderson, C., Hsiung, G. D., and Tenser, R. B. The use of temperature sensitivity and selective cell culture system for differentiation of herpes simplex virus types 1 and 2 in a clinical laboratory. *Proc. Soc. Exp. Biol. Med.* 155: 118, 1977.

Stalder, H., Oxman, M. N., and Herrmann, K. L. Herpes simplex virus microneutralization: a simplification of the test. *J. Infect. Dis.* 131: 423, 1975.

Whitley, R. J., Soong, S. J., Dolin, R., et al. Adenine arabinoside therapy of biopsy-proved herpes simplex encephalitis. *N. Eng. J. Med.* 297: 289, 1977.

Cytomegalovirus

Review Papers

Hanshaw, J. B. Cytomegalovirus. Virology Monogr. 3: 1, 1968.

Weller, T. H. The cytomegaloviruses: ubiquitous agents with protean clinical manifestations. *N. Eng. J. Med.* 285: 203, 267, 1971.

Specific Articles

Booth, J. C., Hannington, G., Aziz, T. A., and Stern, H. Comparison of enzyme-linked immunosorbent assay (ELISA) technique and complement-fixation test for estimation of cytomegalovirus IgG antibody. *J. Clin. Path.* 32: 122, 1979.

Cremer, N. E., Hoffman, M., and Lennette, E. H. Analysis of antibody assay methods and classes of viral antibodies in serodiagnosis of cytomegalovirus infection. *J. Clin. Micro.* 8: 152, 1978.

Cremer, N. E., Hoffman, M., and Lennette, E. H. Role of rheumatoid factor in complement-fixation and indirect hemagglutination tests for immunoglobulin M antibody to cytomegalovirus. *J. Clin. Micro.* 8: 160, 1978.

Keller, R. R., Peitchel, R., Goldman, J. N., and Goldman, M. An IgG-Fc receptor induced in cytomegalovirus infected human fibroblasts. *J. Immun.* 116: 772, 1976.

Lee, F. K., Nahmias, A. J., and Stagno, S. Rapid diagnosis of cytomegalovirus infection in infants by electron microscopy. *N. Eng. J. Med.* 299: 1266, 1978.

Swack, N. S., Michalski, F. J., Baumgarten, A., and Hsiung, G. D. Indirect fluorescent-antibody test for human cytomegalovirus infection in the absence of interfering immunoglobulin G receptors. *Infect. Immun.* 16: 522, 1977.

Varicella-Zoster Virus

Specific Articles

Almeida, J. D., Howatson, H. F., and Williams, M. Morphology of varicella (chicken pox) virus. *Virology* 16: 353, 1962.

Forghani, B., Schmidt, N. J., and Dennis, J. Antibody assay for varicella-zoster virus: comparison of enzyme immunoassay with neutralization, immune adherence hemagglutination and complement fixation. *J. Clin. Micro.* 8: 545, 1978.

Germa, G., and Chambers, R. W. Varicella-zoster plaque assay and plaque reduction neutralization test by the immunoperoxidase technique. *J. Clin. Micro.* 4: 437, 1976.

Weller, T. H., Witton, M. M., and Bell, E. J. The etiologic agents of varicella and herpes zoster: isolation, propagation and cultural characteristics in vitro. *J. Exp. Med.* 108: 843, 1958.

Epstein-Barr Virus

Books and Review Papers

Henle, W., Henle, G., and Horwitz, C. A. Infectious mononucleosis and Epstein-Barr virus associated malignancies. In *Diagnostic procedures for viral, rickettsial and chlamydial infections*, ed. E. H. Lennette and N. J. Schmidt, p. 441. 5th ed. Washington, D.C.: American Public Health Association, 1979.

Miller, G. The oncogenicity of Epstein-Barr virus. *J. Infect. Dis.* 130: 187, 1974.

Specific Articles

Diehl, V., Henle, G., Henle, W., and Kohn G. Demonstration of a herpes group virus in cultures of peripheral leukocytes from patients with infectious mononucleosis. *J. Virol.* 2: 663, 1968.

Epstein, M. A., Achong, B. G., and Barr, Y. M. Virus particles in cultured lymphoblasts from Burkitt's lymphoma. *Lancet* 1: 702, 1964.

Henle, G., Henle, W., and Horwitz, C. A. Antibodies to Epstein-Barr virus associated nuclear antigens in infectious mononucleosis. *J. Infect. Dis.* 130: 231, 1974.

Henle, W., Henle, G., and Zajae, B. A. Differential reactivity of human serums with early antigens induced by Epstein-Barr virus. *Science* 169: 188, 1970.

Henle, W., Ho, H. C., Henle, G., Chang, J. C. W., and Kwang, H. C. Nasopharyngeal carcinoma: significance of changes in Epstein-Barr virus related antibody patterns following therapy. *Int. J. Cancer* 20: 663, 1977.

Miller, G., Niederman, J. C., and Andrew, L. Prolonged oropharyngeal excretion of EB virus after infectious mononucleosis. *N. Eng. J. Med.* 288: 229, 1973.

Robinson, J. E., Smith, D., and Niederman, J. Plasmacytic differentiation of circulating Epstein-Barr virus infected B lymphocytes during infectious mononucleosis. *J. Exp. Med.* 153: 235, 1981.

21. Poxviridae

VARIOLA AND VACCINIA VIRUSES

Three serologically indistinguishable poxviruses—vaccinia, variola major (smallpox), and variola minor (alastrim)—are associated with different forms of human disease. The alastrim virus is considerably less virulent than the virus of smallpox, which has now been eradicated in most parts of the world. Vaccinia virus is not, in general, highly pathogenic for man, although it may produce severe generalized infection following vaccination and, in rare instances, ocular infection. Infection of humans by monkey poxvirus is indistinguishable from that by variola; most patients are not severely ill although 6 deaths have been reported in association with exposure to the virus.

Morphologically, all poxviruses are similar in shape and structure: they are brick-shaped and large in size, 230 × 300 nm. Virus particles of this group can be easily recognized in crust extracts or in vesicle fluids by means of electron microscopy. Similarly, large numbers of poxvirus particles were often observed in biopsy tissues obtained from molluscum contagiosum (figure 87). Vaccinia virus can be propagated in a variety of cell culture systems and a large number of similar pox virus particles are seen in an infected cell (figure 88).

Poxvirus induces eosinophilic cytoplasmic inclusions or Guarnieri bodies in infected cells. Following light microscopic examination of stained smears obtained from skin or mucous membrane lesions, virus particles or elementary bodies can be seen. This direct method was first used by Paschen in 1906 and has been of great diagnostic value since that time. The viruses are stable even at room temperature for several months, and refrigeration is not necessary when specimens for virus isolation are shipped by mail. Unlike the vaccinia virus, infection with variola is restricted to man and monkey. In the laboratory, CAM of embryonated chicken eggs are highly susceptible, thus inoculation of the latter is still the most reliable laboratory test for the detection of this group of viruses. More recently, Vero cell culture and human diploid fibroblasts (HDF)

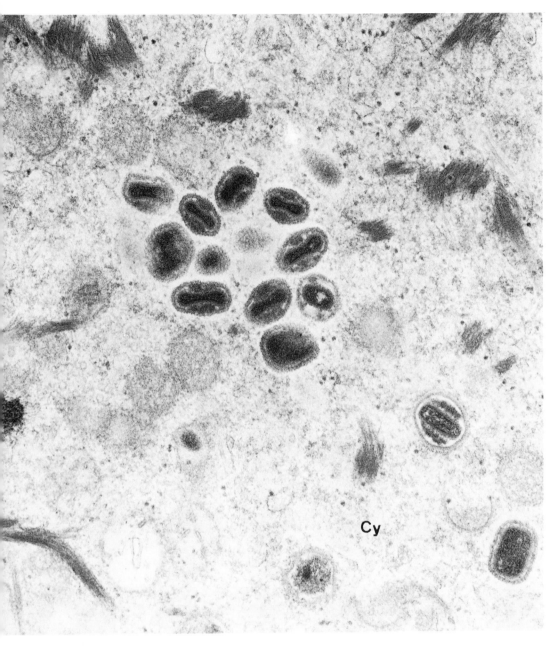

Figure 87. Electron micrograph of poxvirus particles in the cytoplasm (Cy) of a cell from molluscum contagiosum tissue (48,000X).

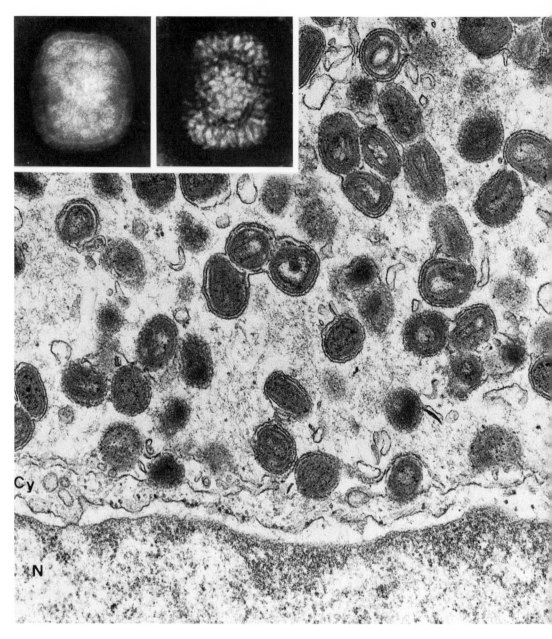

Figure 88. Electron micrographs of vaccinia virus in an infected RhMK cell, showing many poxvirus particles in the cytoplasmic inclusion (48,000X). N = nucleus; Cy = cytoplasm. Insets: Vaccinia virus particles stained with PTA showing different appearance of virus structure (100,800X) (modified from C. K. Y. Fong and G. D. Hsiung, in *Virology and rickettsiology*, vol. 1, pt. 1, p. 99).

have been found useful for the propagation of variola, vaccinia, and monkey poxviruses.

Specimen Inoculation

Scrapings from skin lesions and vesicle fluids and crusts are good sources for virus isolation. These can be inoculated directly onto the CAM of 12- to 14-day-old embryonated chicken eggs. Monkey kidney, Hep-2, and a variety of other cells are also susceptible to vaccinia virus infection.

Virus Isolation, Propagation, and Assay

Cytopathic effect in fluid cultures. Vaccinia virus produces CPE in a variety of cell cultures of both primary and passaged cell lines within 18 to 24 hours of infection. Cytopathic effect induced by vaccinia virus in Hep-2 (figure 89) and RhMK cells (figure 90) is characterized by multinucleated giant cells. Extensive distortion of the monolayers is typical of vaccinia virus infection. Eosinophilic cytoplasmic inclusions are easily distinguishable in the infected RhMK cells (figure 91). These inclusions are Feulgen-positive, indicating the presence of DNA.

Pock formation on CAM of embryonated eggs. Inoculation of the CAM of embryonated chicken eggs is the most reliable laboratory test for the isolation of the poxviruses. Embryos 12- to 14-days old are most suitable for propagation; virus pocks appear in 2 to 3 days. Variola and vaccinia virus can be distinguished by differences in size and morphology of pocks produced on the CAM of embryonated chicken eggs (figure 92). The pocks produced by variola virus are small whereas the vaccinia virus pocks are large and ulcerated.

Animal pathogenicity. Vaccinia virus readily produces lesions on the skin of rabbits and kills infant mice after intracerebral inoculation; variola virus is nonpathogenic for these animal species (table 24).

Plaque formation. Vaccinia virus induces plaques in cultures with liquid medium as well as under agar overlay medium (figure 93). Distinct virus-induced plaques that usually appear 3–6 days after inoculation are commonly used as a tool for virus assay.

Identification of Isolates

An early presumptive diagnosis of poxvirus infection can be made most rapidly by observing virus particles in negatively stained preparations of vesicle fluid under EM examination. Virus particles, i.e. elementary bodies, in a Giemsa-stained smear of scrapings from the base of skin lesions can also be easily recognized. Smears from skin lesions or vesicle fluid can be stained by the IF technique with immune serum to vaccinia virus. Better results are obtained with cultured cells that have been infected with the isolate for 16 to 24 hours, followed by the IF staining technique. Poxvirus strains can be differentiated by

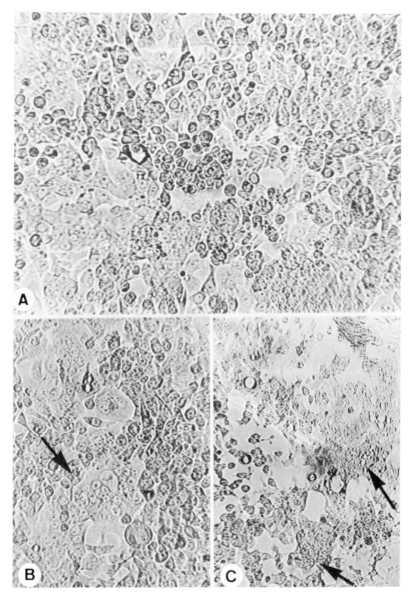

Figure 89. Cytopathic effect (CPE) induced by vaccinia virus in Hep-2 cell cultures (100X).
  A. Uninfected Hep-2 culture.
  B. Early CPE; note area of multinucleated cells (arrow).
  C. Late CPE; note area of multinucleated cells (arrows).

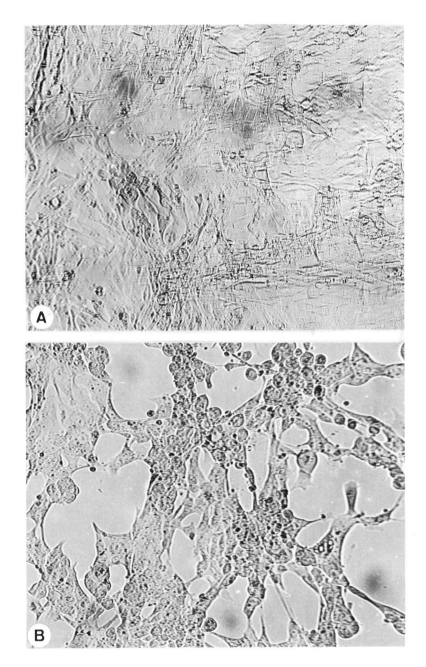

Figure 90. Cytopathic effect (CPE) induced by vaccinia virus in RhMK cell cultures (100X).
    A. RhMK cell culture control.
    B. CPE induced by vaccinia virus.

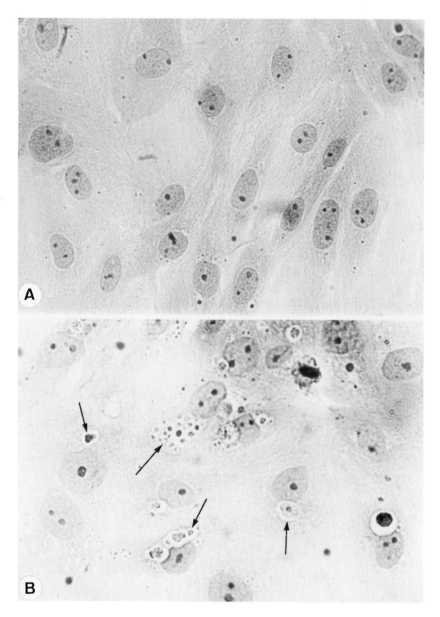

Figure 91. Eosinophilic intracytoplasmic inclusions induced by vaccinia virus in RhMK cell cultures (H&E, 400X).
    A. Uninfected RhMK culture.
    B. Eosinophilic intracytoplasmic inclusions (arrows) in RhMK cells.

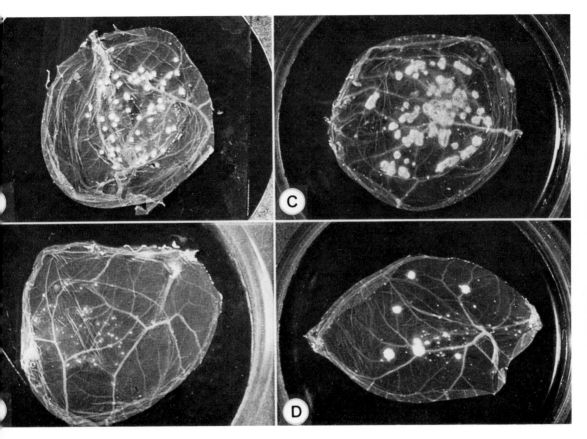

Figure 92. Pock formation with variola and vaccinia viruses on CAM of embryonated eggs
(K. R. Dumbell, *Progr. med. Virol.* 10: 394, 1968).
A. Variola major, 3 days at 35°C.
B. Variola major, 3 days at 38.2°C; note small size of pocks as compared with (A).
C. Vaccinia virus, 3 days at 35°C; note ulcerated pocks.
D. Pocks are similar to those in (C); shown are small secondary pocks when a lower
   dosage is used.

Table 24. Differential Characteristics of Herpes Simplex, Varicella-Zoster, Vaccinia, and Variola Viruses

Virus Group	Virus Type	Direct Examination of Smears or Scrapings	Reaction to 20°C Temperature	Tissue Culture				Pocks on Chorioallantoic Membrane	Effect of Inoculation on Mice or Rabbits
				CPE			Inclusion Bodies		
				MK	HDF	Hep-2			
Herpes	Herpes Simplex	multinucleated giant cells with intranuclear inclusions	labile	+/-	+	+	intranuclear inclusions (Cowdry type A)	pinpoint for type 1; large, clear for type 2	death
	Varicella-Zoster	multinucleated giant cells with intranuclear inclusions	labile	-	+[a]	-	intranuclear inclusions (Cowdry type A)	none	no effect
Pox	Variola	elementary bodies (virus particles)	stable	+/-	+/-	+/-	intracytoplasmic inclusions (Guarnieri bodies)	small, discreet, circular	no effect
	Vaccinia	elementary bodies (virus particles)	stable	+	+	+	intracytoplasmic inclusions (Guarnieri bodies)	large, diffused, hemorrhagic, necrotic	death or lesions

[a]Tissue cells from human embryonic lung or skin are preferable, and infectious virus material is best passaged serially from infected cells.

Key: + = virus-induced change
     - = no change

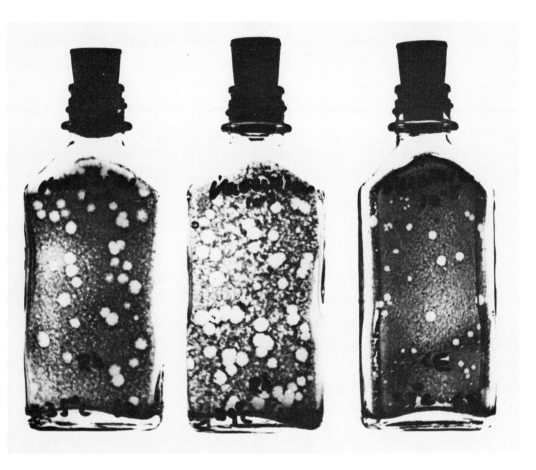

Figure 93. Plaque formation of vaccinia virus in RhMK and chicken embryo (CE) fibroblast cell cultures. RhMK cell cultures incubated at 35°C (bottle at left) and 39°C (center bottles); CE fibroblast culture (bottle at right) incubated at 37°C, 6 days after inoculation.

pock morphology on CAM (figure 92); variola pocks are small and discrete, whereas vaccinia virus pocks are diffused and necrotic.

Variola and vaccinia virus can also be differentiated by their temperature sensitivity. Variola and alastrim viruses do not produce pocks on the CAM when the eggs are incubated at 39°C to 40°C. Alastrim does not produce pocks on CAM at or above 38°C, whereas variola virus produces small-sized pocks at 38.2°C (figure 92). Vaccinia virus induces pocks on the CAM of embryonated eggs incubated at both 35°C and 38.5°C.

The final identification of poxvirus isolates may be made by immunofluorescence or CF test. However, a specific type of variola, alastrim, or vaccinia virus cannot be identified because of the serologic relationships within the poxvirus group.

Differentiation of herpes simplex, varicella-zoster, vaccinia, and variola viruses (table 24). Since herpes simplex virus and vaccinia virus occasionally cause severe generalized vesicular eruptions in individuals with atopic eczema and, rarely, varicella-zoster virus may do the same, isolation of the virus in cell culture for purposes of identification is important. When facilities are available, electron microscopic examination of negatively stained preparations of lesion fluid can permit the diagnosis within hours, since herpes virus and poxvirus particles are easily distinguished from each other (figure 71 inset and figure 88 inset). Indirect immonofluorescent staining technique using specific antiserum to each virus type is the most useful and rapid method for distinguishing HSV, VZV, and vaccinia virus infection in cells taken from lesions. Under these circumstances other useful biologic properties that can be compared include the type of pock produced on the CAM of chick embryos, pathogenicity in mice and rabbits, and the type of inclusion produced in infected cells, each of which is specifically characteristic of each virus (table 24).

Electron microscopy. The diagnosis of poxvirus infection following negative staining of vesicle fluids has been used for over 30 years and is a well-established diagnostic procedure. Rapid diagnosis of smallpox is extremely important from a public-health point of view. Use of this technique is common as a means to distinguish between poxvirus and herpes-virus in skin lesions.

Serodiagnosis

Serologic methods are not suitable for quick and accurate diagnosis of smallpox virus infection. However, when no specimen is available for virologic studies, a 4-fold rise in antibody titer can be measured by CF or neutralization tests. Neutralizing antibody titers may persist for years whereas the CF antibody titers are usually detectable for only 6 to 8 months after vaccination with vaccinia virus.

SUPPLEMENTARY READING

Books and Review Papers

Dowdle, W. R. Exotic viral diseases. *Yale J. Biol. Med.* 53: 109, 1980.

Nakano, J. H. Smallpox, monkeypox, vaccinia, and whitepox viruses. In *Manual of clinical microbiology*, ed. E. H. Lennette et al., p. 810. 3rd ed. Washington, D. C.: American Society for Microbiology, 1980.

Specific Articles

Arita, I. Virological evidence for the success of the smallpox eradication programme. *Nature* 279: 293, 1979.

Cruickshank, J. G., Bedson, H. S., and Watson, D. H. Electron microscopy in the rapid diagnosis of small pox. *Lancet* 2: 527, 1966.

Dumbell, J. R. Laboratory aids to the control of smallpox in countries where the disease is not endemic. *Progr. Med. Virol.* 10: 388, 1968.

Williams, M. G., Almeida, J. D., and Howatson, A. F. Electron microscope studies on viral skin lesions: a simple and rapid method of identifying virus particles. *Arch. Dermatol.* 86: 290, 1962.

World Health Organization. Guide to the laboratory diagnosis of smallpox for smallpox eradication programmes. Geneva: World Health Organization, 1969.

22. Papovaviridae

WART, BK, AND JC VIRUSES

The name papovavirus was originally derived from three groups of viruses, the human papillomavirus, mouse polyomavirus, and the vacuolating virus of monkeys. Although this group of viruses has not been associated with any of the acute, highly infectious disease syndromes that are of concern to the clinician, increasing evidence of an association between some papovaviruses and the slow virus diseases of humans, as well as the finding of papovavirus excretion in the urine of immunosuppressed patients, increases the importance of these viruses in clinical medicine.

The papovaviruses are generally grouped into two major subgroups: the papillomaviruses and the polyomaviruses (table 25). In humans the most commonly encountered member is the human papilloma (wart) virus. Its causal association with the development and spread of warts is well documented. More recently, the JC virus has been encountered in association with progressive multifocal leukoencephalopathy (PML) and the BK virus has been isolated from patients under immunosuppressive therapy.

Morphologically, the papillomaviruses (figure 94) are slightly larger (50–55 nm in diameter) than polyomaviruses, which are 40–45 nm in diameter (figures 95 and 96). In negatively stained samples, papovavirus particles appear as nonenveloped viruses consisting of double-stranded DNA enclosed in an icosahedral nucleocapsid composed of 72 capsomeres. In a thin section of an infected cell, numerous virus particles can be seen scattered throughout the nucleus (figures 95 and 96A). These viruses are very stable and are resistant to ether treatment.

Specimen Inoculation

Brain biopsy samples from PML patients are used for isolation of JC virus by cocultivation method; urine samples obtained from immunosuppressed patients are inoculated into human fibroblast cells for BK virus isolation.

Table 25. Representative Papovaviruses

Virus Group	Virus Type Commonly Known	Source of Virus Specimens
Papilloma	human papilloma virus	human (wart)
	rabbit papilloma virus	rabbit
	bovine papilloma virus	cattle
	canine papilloma virus	dog
	hamster papilloma virus	hamster
Polyoma	human JC virus	human brain
	human BK virus	urine from immunosuppressed patient
	simian vacuolating virus (SV_{40})	monkey kidney
	mouse polyoma virus	mouse tissue
	mouse K virus	mouse

Virus Isolation, Propagation, and Assay

Characteristic intranuclear inclusions in scrapings of wart tissue or biopsy materials are easily recognized. However, isolation of papovavirus requires exceedingly prolonged cultivation of tissue cells or cocultivation of infected cells with human embryonic cells. Therefore, it is not commonly done in a routine diagnostic virology laboratory, although increased demands for isolation of BK virus from urine of immunosuppressed patients exists. Electron microscopic examination of urine or tissue suspected of harboring virus can provide evidence of the presence of members of this group.

Electron microscopy. The wart viruses are not commonly isolated by the conventional tissue culture methods. In addition to clinical diagnosis, direct visualization of virus particles in clinical specimens by either negative staining or by thin-sectioning techniques are convincing evidence of human papillomavirus infection. Figure 94 illustrates a thin section of a human skin tumor showing papillomavirus particles in aggregate in an infected nucleus. An example of an unidentified human polyomavirus isolated from the urine of an immunosuppressed patient grown in cell culture is illustrated in figure 95. Virus particles are usually scattered in the nucleus of the infected cells. Negatively stained particles of the same sample are shown in the inset (figure 95). Although SV_{40} is not a human virus, it is often present in primary rhesus monkey kidney cell cultures as a source of endogenous virus contamination. Therefore it is important to recognize its presence. For comparison, an example of SV_{40} in monkey kidney cells is illustrated in figure 96.

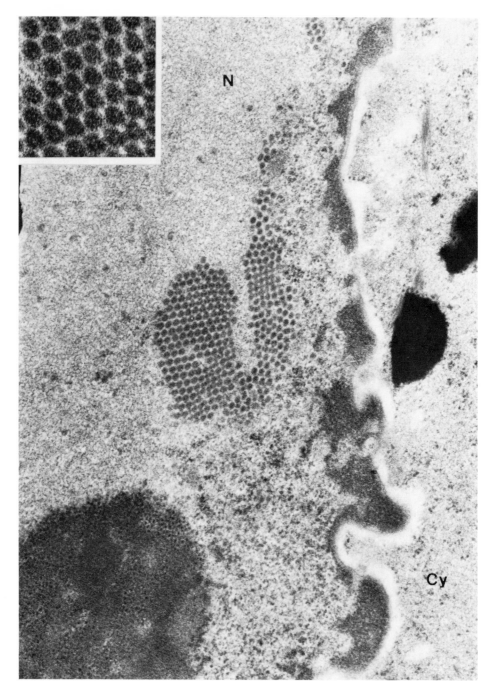

Figure 94. Electron micrograph of human papillomavirus particles in the nucleus of a cell from a wart (38,400X). Inset: Higher magnification of the viral aggregate (108,900X) (courtesy of S. Klaus).

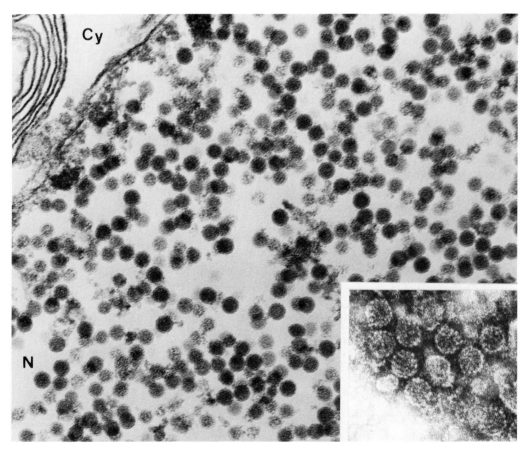

Figure 95. Electron micrograph of human papovavirus isolated from a urine sample that was inoculated into HDF cell culture; N = nucleus, Cy = cytoplasm (100,800X). Inset: Same virus particles stained with PTA (168,000X) (original specimen supplied by M. Hirsch, Harvard Medical School).

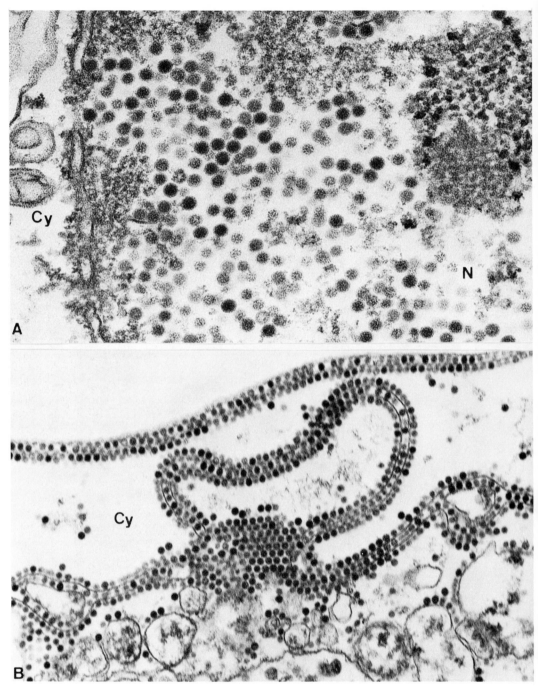

Figure 96. Electron micrographs of simian papovavirus, SV_{40}, in an African green monkey kidney cell (C. K. Y. Fong and G. D. Hsiung, in *Virology and rickettsiology*, vol. 1, pt. 1, p. 84).

A. Virus particles in the nucleus (N); CY = cytoplasm (88,000X).

B. Virus particles in association with membranes of a disrupted cell (48,000X).

SUPPLEMENTARY READING

Review Papers

Oxman, M. N. Papovaviridae. In *Virology and rickettsiology*, ed. G. D. Hsiung and R. H. Green, vol. 1, pt. 2, p. 17. Handbook series in clinical laboratory science, Section H. West Palm Beach, Fla.: CRC Press, 1978.

Takemoto, K. K. Human papovaviruses. *Int. Rev. Exp. Pathol.* 18: 281, 1978.

Specific Articles

Coleman, D. V., Russell, W. J., Hodgson, J., Pe, T., and Mowbray, J. F. Human papovavirus in Papanicolaou smears of urinary sediment detected by transmission electron microscopy. *J. Clin. Pathol.* 30: 1015, 1977.

Gardner, S. D., Field, A. M., Coleman, D. V., and Huline, B. New human papovirus (B.K.) isolated from urine after renal transplantation. *Lancet* 1: 1253, 1971.

Lecatsas, G., Prozesky, O. W., Van Wyk, J., and Els, H. J. Papovavirus in urine after renal transplantation. *Nature* 241: 343, 1973.

Padgett, B. L., Walker, D. L., ZuRhein, G. M., Eckroade, R. J., and Dessel, B. H. Cultivation of papova-like virus from human brain with progressive multifocal leukoencephalopathy. *Lancet* 1: 1257, 1971.

Padgett, B. L., Walker, D. L., ZuRhein, G. M., Hodach, A. E., and Chou, S. M. JC papovavirus in progressive multifocal leukoencephalopathy. *J. Infect. Dis.* 133: 686, 1976.

UNCLASSIFIED VIRUSES

23. Hepatitis Viruses

The nature of hepatitis, characterized by the jaundiced appearance of the patient, was recognized as early as the seventeenth century. However, the separate disease entities of infectious hepatitis and serum hepatitis, each caused by a different infectious agent with distinctly different epidemiologic patterns, have only been reported since the 1940s. Each disease has a different mode of transmission and incubation period (table 26). At present there are at least three distinct groups of viruses responsible for hepatitis: hepatitis A virus (HAV), hepatitis B virus (HBV), and an uncharacterized group of viruses referred to as non-A, non-B hepatitis or hepatitis C viruses.

The recognition of hepatitis B virus was first made by Blumberg, when testing the serum of an Australian aborigine, which he described as the Australia antigen and is now termed hepatitis B surface antigen. Subsequently, Dane et al. observed in serum from patients with serum hepatitis a 42-nm viruslike particle together with other small particles and filamentous forms (figure 97). Thus, HBV particles exhibit three distinct structures: the Dane particle, 42 nm in diameter with an electron-dense DNA-containing core (HBc); and the surface antigen (HBsAg), either a small spherical particle, with an average diameter of about 22 nm (the most numerous), or a filamentous form, about 22 nm in diameter and ranging in length from 50 nm to greater than 200 nm. The Dane particles are the infectious virus particles.

Hepatitis A virus, a highly infectious agent, has now been identified by immunoelectron microscopy (IEM) as a 27-nm viruslike particle present in filtrates of acute-phase stool samples from patients with infectious viral hepatitis (figure 98). The hepatitis A virus is believed to contain RNA, suggesting a possible classification with the picornaviridae. It is acid- and ether-stable and relatively heat-resistant.

Table 26. Differences between Hepatitis A and Hepatitis B

Properties	Hepatitis A	Hepatitis B
Traditional name	infectious hepatitis	serum hepatitis
Major mode of transmission	fecal-oral	parenteral inoculation
Incubation period	15–40 days	60–160 days
Virus name	hepatitis A virus (HAV)	hepatitis B virus (HBV)
Source of virus	Feces	blood (serum) (less common in feces, urine)
Virus nucleic acid	RNA	DNA
Virus particle size and physical traits	27-nm, naked particle	42-nm double-enveloped Dane particle (28-nm inner core and 7-nm outer envelope); 22-nm surface antigen, spherical and filamentous in form
Major serologic tests		
Immunoelectron microscopy	virus particles in feces	virus particles in serum or liver biopsy extracts
Immunofluorescent or immunoperoxidase staining	liver biopsy	liver biopsy
Complement-fixation, radioimmunoassay, or ELISA	detection of HAV antigen or antibody	detection of HBV surface antigen, antibody to surface antigen, or antibody to core antigen

Clinical, Epidemiological, and Serological Markers

Hepatitis A. The onset of hepatitis A is usually sudden after an incubation period of 15–40 days. It generally occurs in individuals with a history of contact with jaundiced persons or contact with contaminated food or water. Primary antibody response to hepatitis A virus, i.e., anti-HAV IgM, usually coincides with the appearance of clinical symptoms and thus serves as the best serological marker for a recent acute HAV infection. On the other hand, the presence of only anti-HAV IgG confirms past hepatitis A infections and suggests probable immunity.

Hepatitis B. The onset of hepatitis B is insidious with a long incubation period, 60–160 days. Rash and arthralgia are sometimes observed. The disease usually occurs in patients receiving blood products or those exposed by needle sticks or cuts from contaminated glassware.

Patients with hepatitis B infection are expected to have three or more marker responses during the course of infection: (1) the presence of HBsAg, (2) the appearance of anti-HBc (core antibody), shortly after the appearance of HBsAg, that usually persists for a life-time, and (3) the appearance of anti-HBs 2–16

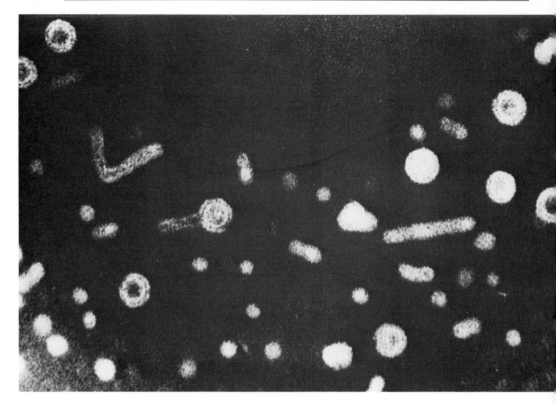

Figure 97. Electron micrograph of hepatitis B virus particles in a serum sample following PTA
staining. Dane particles, surface antigen, both 22-nm spherical particles and filamentous forms are present (220,000X).

weeks after HBsAg is no longer detectable, and/or (4) the presence of anti-HBc
in the absence of HBsAg and anti-HBs, which is a good indication of a recent
HBV infection. The presence of another antigen, HBeAg, in HBsAg-positive
serum suggests that the serum is likely to be infectious.

Specimens to be Tested

Stool, serum, and/or liver biopsy specimens are used for diagnosis of hepatitis
virus infection either by electron microscopy or by serological tests for the
various markers mentioned above.

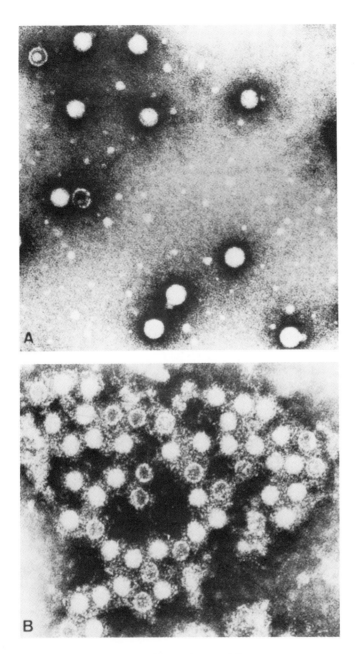

Figure 98. Electron micrographs of hepatitis A virus particles.
    A. Stool sample following purification and PTA staining, showing hepatitis A virus
        particles (150,000X) (reproduced from H. Ginsberg, in *Virology*, ed. R. Dulbecco
        and H. S. Ginsberg, Harperstown, Md.: Harper & Row, 1980, p. 1219).
    B. IEM of liver extract following PTA staining. Note aggregates containing full and
        empty virus particles (reproduced from J. L. Dienstag and R. H. Purcell, in
        Virology and rickettsiology, vol. 1, pt. 2, p. 164).

Virus Isolation, Propagation, and Assay

Isolation and cultivation of hepatitis A virus in cell cultures is currently done only in research laboratories and not in diagnostic laboratories. Both A and B viruses can infect chimpanzees and monkeys and each virus can be identified by electron microscopy. However, because of the distinct immunologic responses of each virus type as stated above, differential diagnosis of hepatitis A and B virus infections using various serologic markers is widely applied. There are no serologic markers specific for non-A, non-B hepatitis, which is diagnosed by exclusion.

Serodiagnosis

Serologic tests provide the most sensitive and economic means for detecting hepatitis viral antigens and/or antibodies. The immunofluorescent technique has been used to identify HAV or HBV in liver biopsy. Other serologic tests, including immune adherence hemagglutination, complement-fixation, solid-phase RIA, ELISA, and several others, are used but the RIA is the most sensitive for detection of either antigen or antibody. Commercial reagents are available and have been used extensively for screening, especially of blood donors. The differential diagnosis of patients with acute viral hepatitis is outlined in table 27.

Electron microscopy. Immunoelectron microscopy has been used for identifying virus particles of HAV in stool samples (figure 98B). Occasionally HAV particles are seen in stool filtrate without the need of special procedures (figure 98A). Hepatitis B surface antigen and Dane particles in serum specimens can be differentiated by direct examination of negatively stained preparations (figure

Table 27. Differential Serodiagnoses of Acute Viral Hepatitis

Anti-HAV IgM	Test Result HBsAg	Anti-HBc	Interpretation
+	−	−	recent acute hepatitis A infection
−	+	−	early acute hepatitis B infection
−	+	+	acute hepatitis B infection or chronic carrier
−	−	+	possible recent hepatitis B infection
−	−	−	possible non-A, non-B hepatitis infection, or other viral infection
+	+	+	recent probable hepatitis A infection and probable chronic hepatitis B infection or chronic carrier

Key: + = virus-induced change
     − = no change

97). Similarly, hepatitis B virus–particle aggregates also can be visualized under EM following treatment either with anti-HBs or anti-HBc. Thus EM and IEM provide a major tool for firm diagnosis of hepatitis A or B virus infection, in addition to the various serologic tests mentioned above.

SUPPLEMENTARY READING

Review Papers

Dienhardt, F. Medical perspectives: predictive value of markers of hepatitis infection. *J. Infect. Dis.* 141: 299, 1980.

Dienstag, J. L. Hepatitis viruses: characterization and diagnostic techniques. *Yale J. Biol. Med.* 53: 61, 1980.

LeBouvier, G. L., and McCollum, R. W. Australia (hepatitis-associated) antigen: physiochemical and immunological characteristics. *Adv. Virus Res.* 16: 357, 1970.

Melnick, J. L., Dressman, G. R., and Hollinger, F. B. Approaching the control of viral hepatitis type B. *J. Infect. Dis.* 133: 210, 1976.

Purcell, R. H. The viral hepatitides. *Hospital Practice* 131: 51, 1978.

Specific Articles

Blumberg, B. S., Alter, H. S., and Visnich, S. A. A "new" antigen in leukemia sera. *JAMA* 191: 541, 1965.

Bradley, D. W., Fields, H. A., McCaustland, K. A., Maynard, J. E., Decker, R. H., Whillington, R., and Overby, L. R. Serodiagnosis of viral hepatitis A by a modified competitive binding radioimmunoassay for immunoglobulin M anti-hepatitis A virus. *J. Clin. Microl.* 9: 120, 1979.

Dane, D. S., Cameron, C. H., and Briggs, M. Virus-like particles in serum of patients with Australia-antigen-associated hepatitis. *Lancet* 1: 695, 1970.

Krugman, S., Overby, L. R., Mushahwar, I. K., Ling, C-M., Frosner, G. G., and Deinhardt, M. C. Viral hepatitis, type B: studies on natural history and prevention re-examined. *N. Engl. J. Med.* 300: 101, 1979.

Mathieson, L. R., Fienstone, S. M., Wong, D. C., Skinboej, P., and Purcell, R. H. Enzyme-linked immunosorbent assay for detection of hepatitis A antigen in stool and antibody to hepatitis A in sera: comparison with solid-phase radioimmunoassay, immune electron microscopy and immune adherence hemagglutination assay. *J. Clin. Microbiol.* 7: 184, 1978.

Provost, P. J., and Hilleman, M. R. Propagation of human hepatitis A virus in cell culture in vitro. *Proc. Soc. Exp. Biol. Med.* 160: 213, 1979.

Siegl, G., and Frosner, G. G. Characterization and classification of virus particles associated with hepatitis A. 1. Size, density and sedimentation. *J. Virology* 26: 40, 1978.

Summer, J., Smolec, J. M., and Snyder, R. A virus similar to human hepatitis B virus associated with hepatitis and hepatoma in woodchucks. *Proc. Nat. Acad. Sci. U.S.A.* 75: 4533, 1978.

WHO Expert Committee on Viral Hepatitis. Terminology of hepatitis viruses and antigens. *Intervirology* 8: 65, 1977.

PART 4: Cell Culture

24. Cell Culture Preparation

The technique of cultivating animal cells in monolayers on glass has provided the virologist with an important and versatile tool for isolating many types of viruses of medical importance. As the field has developed it has become apparent that the greater the number and variety of systems used for culture, the greater the number of viruses that can be isolated. In a working diagnostic laboratory, however, it is necessary to limit the number of culture systems used to those most likely to reveal pathogenic agents. Which culture system to employ routinely depends upon a number of factors, including individual preferences based on experience. The availability of animal tissues for primary cultures and the size and capacity to maintain different serial cell lines in the laboratory are also important determinants. In general, a primary monkey kidney cell culture, a human diploid cell strain, and/or a human cell line such as HeLa or Hep-2 constitute a satisfactory combination. Primary human kidney, human amnion, or other human diploid cell lines may be used if readily available. A summary of the different cell systems applicable to the different groups of viruses is listed in table 2.

The criteria for recognition of potential virus isolates in cell culture may not always include cytopathic effects and/or plaque formation. The inducement of cytopathology in cell culture during virus multiplication may depend wholly or in part on such conditions as the multiplicity of virus infection, the strain of virus, the age of the cell culture, the medium in which the cells have been grown, and the medium in which the infected cells are maintained. In some instances, CPE may be unrecognized in cultures with liquid medium while the same infected cultures, under agar overlay medium, may support plaque formation. Supplemental techniques, such as interference, hemadsorption, hemagglutination, and staining techniques, are also used to detect virus replication when the cells in culture show no gross morphologic changes.

False positive virus isolations in cell culture from clinical specimens are relatively uncommon, but there is the possibility that the inoculum might be toxic and produce a nonspecific cytopathology similar to a virus-induced cytopathic effect. In addition, every virus diagnostic laboratory should be aware of the known agents that are considered common contaminants of various cell types. Latent viruses may become activated when animal tissues are subjected to trypsinization and cultured in monolayers. Primary cultures from monkey kidney tissues are probably the most notorious harborers of endogenous virus contaminants. In addition, mycoplasmas are often carried along with passaged cell lines. Such agents may complicate final identification of a suspected isolate obtained from clinical specimens. For this reason it is important to confirm each virus isolate by reisolation in another tissue culture or animal host system.

Cell cultures that are commonly used in a virology laboratory are listed in table 28. Many of these cultures can be purchased commercially. A few of the basic techniques for the preparation of both primary cell cultures and passaged cell lines are listed below. It is imperative that all supplies be sterile.

Table 28. Cell Cultures Commonly Used in a Virology Laboratory

Cell Culture	Common Name	Species Origin	Tissue Origin	Cell Morphology
Primary cell	HEK	human	embryonic kidney	mostly epithelial
	MK	monkey (rhesus, cynomolgus, African green, etc.)	kidney	mostly epithelial
	RK	rabbit	kidney	mostly epithelial
	GPE	guinea pig	whole embryo	mostly fibroblastic
	CE	chicken	whole embryo	mostly fibroblastic
Passaged cell strain or line	HDF[a]	human	lung or foreskin	fibroblastic
	Hep-2	human	carcinoma of larynx	epithelial
	HeLa	human	carcinoma of cervix	epithelial
	KB	human	carcinoma of mouth	epithelial
	Vero	African green monkey	kidney	epithelial
	BSC-1	African green monkey	kidney	epithelial
	RK-13	rabbit	kidney	epithelial
	BHK-21	baby hamster	kidney	fibroblastic
	A549	human	carcinoma of lung	epithelial

[a]Including WI-38, IMR-90, MRC-5; all are diploid cell strains derived from human embryonic lung or foreskin.

Supplies and Equipment

Petri dishes
Scissors
Forceps
Trypsinization flask
Magnetic stirring bar, Teflon-
  or glass-coated
Sterile gauze squares, 4″ × 4″
Funnels
Pipettes, 1, 2, 5, 10 ml

Magnetic stirrer base
Centrifuge bottles, 200 ml
Centrifuge tubes, 15, 50 ml
Rubber stoppers, sizes 0, 00, 2, 6
Graduated cylinders, 50, 100, 250,
  500, 1000 ml
Automatic pipettes, 2, 5, 10 ml
Culture tubes, Leighton tubes
Prescription bottles, 1, 2, 3, 4 oz.
Tissue culture flasks, tissue culture
  plates, and plastic petri dishes

Media and Solutions

1. Trypsin, 0.25%, in PBS + penicillin (200 units per ml) + streptomycin (200 µg per ml). Concentration of trypsin depends upon tissue source.
2. Growth medium, prewarmed to 37°C. Choice of growth medium depends on cell cultures used, usually the minimum essential medium (MEM) with 10% calf serum.
3. Hanks' balanced salt solution (Hanks' BSS).
4. Crystal violet solution for cell counts.

PRIMARY KIDNEY CELL CULTURE

The following method can be adapted for tissues obtained from humans, monkeys, or any animal species. The steps are illustrated in figure 99.

Collection of Tissue

1. Remove kidney aseptically from freshly sacrificed and exsanguinated animal, for example, rabbit or guinea pig.
2. Decapsulate kidney with sterile scissors and forceps; remove connective tissues and blood clots; cut kidneys in half and remove medulla. Wash twice with Hanks' BSS. Cut cortex into small pieces (about 1 mm^3). Transfer cut tissue to a trypsinization flask; wash twice with Hanks' BSS to remove residual blood.

Preparation of Cell Suspension for Culture

3. Add approximately 25 ml prewarmed trypsin (0.25%) to the trypsinization flask and stir with a magnetic stirring bar for 5 minutes. Discard

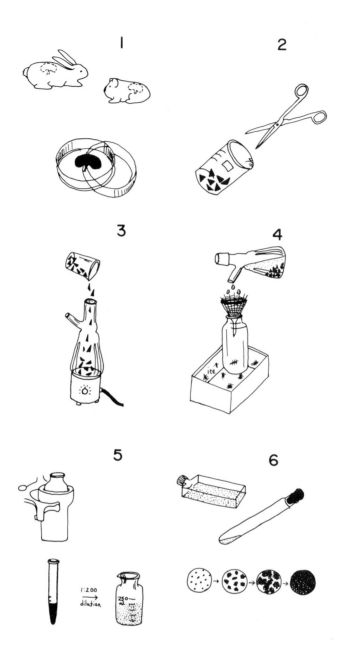

Figure 99. Schematic diagram for preparation of primary kidney cell culture showing equipment and procedures.

first run or keep it separate from subsequent cell suspensions. Add approximately 25–30 ml fresh prewarmed trypsin and stir for 15 minutes.

4. Filter the cell suspension through 2 or 3 layers of sterile gauze. Collect the cell suspension in a 200-ml centrifuge bottle containing approximately 10 ml growth medium; keep cell suspension in an ice bath or refrigerator. Repeat steps 3 and 4 until tissues are exhausted.

5. Centrifuge the cell suspension at 750 rpm for 15 minutes at 4°C; discard supernatant trypsin solution and resuspend the packed cells in growth medium *immediately*, using approximately 30–50 ml for each bottle of packed cells; shake well.

6. Transfer cell suspension into a 50-ml graduated centrifuge tube and recentrifuge at 750 rpm for 10 minutes; discard supernatant; resuspend packed cells with growth medium at 1:200 dilution for rabbit kidney cells, 1:250 dilution for guinea pig kidney cells, and 1:300 for monkey kidney cells.

7. Seed cell suspension 0.5–1.0 ml per tube, 1.5 ml per Leighton tube, 6–9 ml per 3 oz. bottle, etc., by means of automatic or regular pipette.

Note. For more accurate cell counts in the suspension:

1. Add 1 ml crystal violet solution (see p. 270) to 0.5 ml of the cell suspension at Step 5 above; mix well and fill into a hemocytometer counting chamber.

2. Count intact cells in 10 squares of the two chambers (there are 5 squares in each chamber); total number of cells in 10 squares $\times$ 3 $\times$ 10^3 equals total number of cells per milliliter in cell suspension.

3. Adjust cell concentration to 3 $\times$ 10^5 cells per ml with growth medium.

PRIMARY EMBRYO CELL CULTURE

This method can be used for preparation of avian and mammalian embryo cell cultures. However, the concentration of trypsin should be adjusted according to the animal species used. For example, 0.005% trypsin is used for guinea pig embryos and the cells should be removed from the trypsin solution as soon as possible. Otherwise the cells will disintegrate. For avian embryos, a 0.25% trypsin solution is satisfactory.

Collection of Tissue

1. Select chicken embryos 9- to 10-days old, or duck embryos 12- to 14-days old; clean eggshells with 70% ethanol.

2. Open shells over the air sac, remove embryos, decapitate, discard head and feet, and place torsos in a sterile container. Wash torsos in *cold* Hanks' BSS, then mince with scissors.

3. Transfer tissue fragments to a trypsinization flask and wash three times with cold Hanks' BSS to remove blood *as thoroughly as possible*; wash once with prewarmed 0.25% trypsin; add 50–100 ml prewarmed tryspin to the tissue fragments in a trypsinization flask and stir with a magnetic stirring bar for 45 minutes at 37°C (only 5 minutes for GPE cells).
4. Filter cell suspension through six layers of sterile gauze and collect filtrate in a 200-ml centrifuge bottle. Centrifuge at 1000 rpm for 15 minutes; discard trypsin solution, wash cells twice with cold Hanks' BSS, and recentrifuge at 1000 rpm for 15 minutes; discard supernatant. Add 30–40 ml cold Hanks' BSS or growth medium (HLS) to the packed cells and by forced pipetting break the clumps.
5. Refilter cell suspension and collect in a graduated centrifuge tube. Centrifuge at 1000 rpm for 15 minutes and discard the supernatant. Resuspend the packed cells in cold HLS containing 10% calf serum at a 1:10 dilution (1 ml packed cells per 9 ml HLS). The 10% cell suspension can be kept as stock at 4°C for 3–4 days. For seeding, dilute to 1:40 with cold HLS containing 5%–10% calf serum (final concentration, 1:400); seed 6–8 ml per 3-oz. bottle or 1 ml per tube. Incubate cultures at 35°C for 48–72 hours before use.

SERIAL PASSAGED CELL LINES

The subculturing method that follows can be used for other serially passaged cell lines, such as HeLa or KB, as well as for secondary cell cultures. Both primary and passage cell lines can be preserved by the method described below, but the percentage of recovery of primary cells is usually not as good as that of passaged cell lines.

Subculture of Hep-2 Cells

1. Discard supernatant fluid from 7-day-old Hep-2 cell bottle cultures.
2. Add 2 ml trypsin-versene solution (formula, p. 269), prewarmed at 37°C, to each 3-oz. cell culture bottle.
3. Incubate at 37°C for 30–60 seconds.
4. Gently turn bottle over without disturbing the cell sheet; incubate for an additional 2–3 minutes at 37°C.
5. Carefully decant trypsin-versene solution and add 2 ml prewarmed Eagle's growth medium (EHS; p. 267) to suspend the cells.
6. Break the cell clumps by forced pipetting.
7. Prepare a 1:4 dilution of the suspension (for diploid cells make a 1:2 dilution.
8. Seed bottles with 10 ml, tubes with 1 ml, and incubate at 37°C.
9. At 3- to 4-day intervals, replace fluid with Eagle's maintenance medium with 2%–5% calf serum (EES; p. 267).

Preservation of Cells

1. To 0.5 ml packed Hep-2 cells add 8.5 ml of EHS medium and 1 ml of filtered sterile dimethylsulfoxide (DMSO). Distribute into small tubes or ampules, 1 ml per tube.
2. Pack the tubes in an insulated box.
3. Cool box *slowly* in 3 steps:
   a. 4°C for 2 hours.
   b. −20°C for 2 hours or until fluid is frozen.
   c. −70°C for long-term storage either in a regular −70°C freezer or in liquid nitrogen; for the latter, sealed ampules are necessary.
4. Steps 2 and 3 can be simplified if a Nitrofreezer is available.
5. To revive cells from a frozen state:
   a. Defrost cell suspension *rapidly* in a 37°C water bath.
   b. Remove DMSO from cell suspension by centrifugation at 1000 rpm for 10 minutes.
   c. Add Eagle's medium with 10% calf serum to the original 5% cell suspension so that final cell concentration is 0.2%.
   d. Seed 10 ml of this suspension per 3-oz. bottle and incubate at 37°C.
   e. Replace with fresh Eagle's medium (EHS) containing 10% calf serum 24 hours after recovery to remove the DMSO present in the frozen samples.

25. Endogenous Viral Contaminants in Animal Tissues

This chapter provides a brief discussion of certain characteristics of the more common endogenous viral contaminants found in animal cell cultures. It is designed to provide information for recognition of the presence of some of these viral agents.

Uninoculated primary cell cultures made from simian and nonsimian tissues frequently contain viral agents. Because of these endogenous viruses, it is desirable to use germ-free animals or eggs from pathogen-free chicken flocks for tissue culture. The endogenous simian viruses that contaminate primary cell cultures derived from monkeys appear to be the most numerous and comprise a variety of virus types within each virus group. Thus, the following description of simian viruses can be used as a guide for recognizing endogenous viruses present in tissues derived from other animal species.

SIMIAN VIRUSES

The widespread use of tissue cultures prepared from monkey kidneys in the 1960s and 1970s resulted in a large number of reports of endogenous simian viruses recoverable from uninoculated cultures. These viruses, including SV_{40}, SV_5, and foamy viruses, are relatively common and their presence can create problems in the diagnosis of human infection. Table 29 lists the simian virus types that have been reported, although some of them are not necessarily latent.

In the following sections the properties of representative simian viruses from each major virus group are presented as a guide for the recognition of these agents in primary monkey cell cultures. Once a latent infection is recognized, the cultures are considered unsuitable for isolation of virus from clinical specimens.

Table 29. Major Groups of Simian Viruses

Nucleic Acid Type	Size Range[a]	nm	Ether[b] Sensitivity	Virus Group	Simian Virus Type[c]
DNA	Small	< 50	Res.	Papova-	SV_{40}
	Medium	50–100	Res.	Adeno-	Sv_1, SV_{11}, SV_{15}, SV_{17}, SV_{20}, SV_{23}, SV_{25}, SV_{27}, SV_{30-34}, SV_{36-39}, SA_7, SA_{17}, SA_{18}
	Large	> 100	Sens. Res.	Herpes- Pox-	B, M, SA_8, SA_6, CMV, SA_{15} Yaba, monkeypox
RNA	Small	< 50	Res.	Entero-	SV_2, SV_6, SV_{16}, SV_{18}, SV_{26}, SV_{29}, SV_{35}, SV_{42-49}, SA_4
	Medium	50–100	Res.	Reo- Rota-	SV_{12}, SV_{59}, SA_3, SA_{16} SA_{11}
	Large	> 100	Sens.	Myxo- Pseudomyxo- Retro-	SV_5, SV_{41} measles, SA foamy virus types 1–7

[a]See also table 12.
[b]Res. = Resistant; Sens. = Sensitive.
[c]SV = Simian Virus; SA = Simian Agent.

Source: Modified from Hsiung, *Ann. N.Y. Acad. Sci.* 162: 485, 1969.

Simian DNA Viruses

Simian papovavirus. SV_{40}, or the vacuolating virus of monkeys, is one of the most common latent viruses of rhesus monkeys. Cytoplasmic vacuoles characteristic of SV_{40} can be recognized readily when African green monkey, patas monkey, or baboon kidney cell cultures are infected with this virus type (figure 100B1). Difficulties have been encountered with SV_{40}-infected rhesus monkey cells since CPE is not apparent in them. However, with IF staining or in H&E-stained preparations, basophilic intranuclear inclusions can be easily recognized in all infected monkey cells (figure 100B2). Because of its ability to induce tumors in experimental animals, SV_{40} has attracted the interest of many investigators in the field of cancer research for the past decade. Today the molecular biology of SV_{40} genome mapping is well established.

Simian adenoviruses. These viruses are most commonly recovered from rhesus or cynomolgus monkey kidney cultures or from monkey stools. They produce CPE in rhesus monkey kidney cultures that is characterized by rounding and clumping of the cells (figure 100C1). Basophilic intranuclear inclusions are easily identifiable in preparations stained with H&E (figure 100C2). Pin-

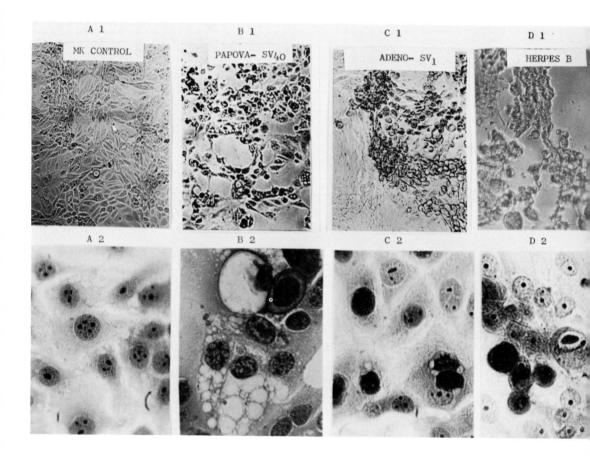

Figure 100. Simian DNA virus–induced cellular changes. Upper row: Simian virus–induced CPE in monkey kidney cells (100X). Lower row: H&E-stained preparations of monkey kidney cells (400X) (G. D. Hsiung, *Bact. Rev.* 32: 192, 1968).

A1, 2. Uninfected RhMK cell cultures.

B1, 2. SV_{40} papovavirus–infected patas MK cells.

C1, 2. SV_1 adenovirus–infected RhMK cells.

D1.   Herpes B virus–infected RhMK cells.

D2.   Monkey cytomegalovirus–infected rhesus monkey cells.

Note intranuclear inclusions in B2, C2, and D2.

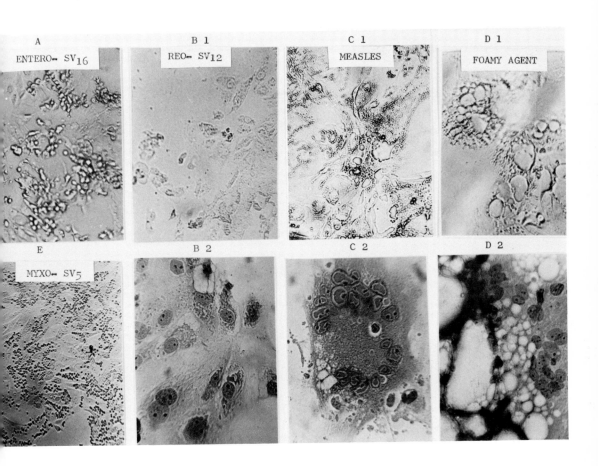

Figure 101. Simian RNA virus–induced cellular changes. Upper row: Simian virus–induced CPE in monkey kidney cell cultures (100X). Lower row: H&E-stained preparations of infected monkey kidney cells (400X, except E, 100X) (G. D. Hsiung, *Bact. Rev.* 32: 193, 1968).

A.   Monkey enterovirus SV_{16}–infected RhMK cells.

B1, 2. Monkey reovirus SV_{12}–infected RhMK cells; note intracytoplasmic inclusions in B2.

C1, 2. Monkey measles virus–infected GMK cells; note intranuclear inclusions in the nuclei of a syncytial cell in C2.

D1, 2. Foamy agent–infected RhMK cells; note absence of intranuclear inclusions in D2.

E.   Monkey parainfluenza virus SV_5-infected RhMK cells; note hemadsorption of guinea pig erythrocytes.

point plaques appear in rhesus and patas monkey kidney cultures 10 to 15 days after inoculation.

Simian herpesvirus. B virus of monkeys is a highly dangerous pathogen for humans although it is of relatively low pathogenicity for rhesus monkeys. B virus can be isolated from the throat, the central nervous system, and the kidney tissues of rhesus monkeys even though no disease is observed in those animals. The virus induces large, rounded clusters of degenerated cells in tissue culture (figure 100D1), and large, clear circular plaques under agar overlay. Monkey cytomegalovirus (CMV) is another member of the simian herpesvirus group. Typical type A intranuclear inclusions are easily recognizable (figure 100D2). Although isolation of monkey CMV does not occur often, high titers of neutralizing antibody to African green monkey CMV is frequently detected in sera collected from green monkeys.

Simian RNA Viruses

Simian enteroviruses. In culture the simian enteroviruses induce CPE characterized by small pleomorphic cells (figure 101A) similar to those induced by human enteroviruses in monkey cells. Simian enteroviruses also produce plaques in monkey kidney bottle cultures. These plaques are large and circular, with islets of healthy stained cells.

Simian reoviruses. Reovirus-infected cells are very granular (figure 101B1); distinct intracytoplasmic eosinophilic inclusions are apparent in stained preparations of infected rhesus cultures (figure 101B2).

Simian pseudomyxoviruses. Monkey measles virus, originally known as MINIA (monkey intranuclear-inclusion agent), produces multinucleated syncytial cells in infected cultures (figure 101C1). In stained preparations, eosinophilic inclusions located in the nuclei as well as in the cytoplasm can be readily seen (figure 101C2).

Simian foamy viruses. These often appear in aged monkey kidney cell cultures, especially in those from rhesus monkey cells. Cytopathic effect takes the form of large vacuoles (figure 101D1), which can be distinguished morphologically from those produced by the vacuolating virus, SV_{40} (figure 100B1). Multiple-nucleated syncytial cells *without* inclusions can be seen in stained cultures (figure 101D2) and can easily be distinguished from measles virus–infected cells in which intranuclear and intracytoplasmic inclusions are present (figure 101C2).

Simian myxovirus. SV_5 is the most common contaminant of kidney cell cultures derived from newly arrived rhesus, cynomolgus, green, and patas monkeys. SV_{41}, serologically related but not identical to SV_5, is also commonly found in green monkey kidney cell cultures. No CPE can be seen in infected cultures, but RBC from various species are easily attached onto SV_5-infected cell sheets (figure 101E). Thus the hemadsorption method is commonly used to detect the presence of these viruses.

Mixed infections. Occasionally a single lot of cell cultures derived from a monkey is infected with two or more virus types. Such mixed infections are

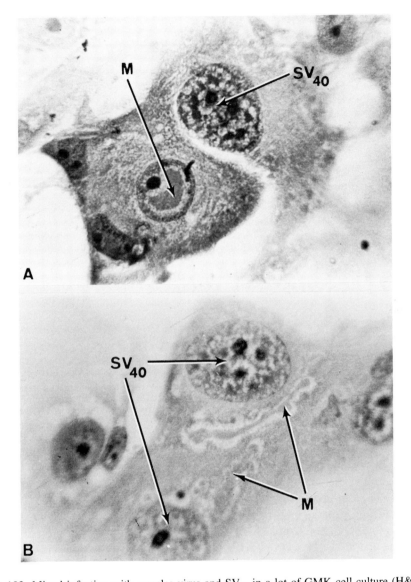

Figure 102. Mixed infection with measles virus and SV_{40} in a lot of GMK cell culture (H&E, 970X) (G. D. Hsiung et al., *Proc. Soc. Exp. Bio. and Med.* 121: 562, 1966).
   A. Measles virus (M) and SV_{40} intranuclear inclusions in two separated cells.
   B. Measles virus (M) intracytoplasmic inclusion and SV_{40} intranuclear inclusions in the same cell.

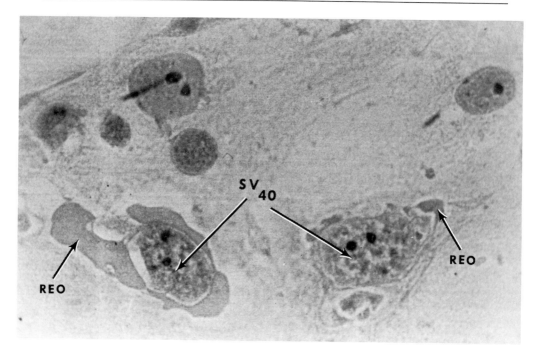

Figure 103. Mixed infection with reovirus and SV_{40} in a lot of GMK cell culture (H&E, 970X). (G. D. Hsiung, *Bact. Rev.* 32: 185, 1968). Intracytoplasmic, eosinophilic inclusion at perinuclear space of reovirus (Reo) and basophilic intranuclear inclusion of SV_{40} are showing in the same cells.

recognized either by light or electron microscopy. Mixed infections of SV_{40} and measles viruses are illustrated in color figure 1 and figure 102. Two distinct types of intranuclear inclusions can be seen in the multinucleated giant cell in which the eosinophilic inclusions are due to measles virus and the basophilic inclusions are due to SV_{40}. Single cells doubly infected with two viruses, for example SV_{40} and measles (figure 102B) or SV_{40} and reovirus (figure 103 and color figure 2), have been observed. Doubly infected cells are easily recognized under EM. Examples are shown in figures 104 and 105. Figure 104 shows measles nucleocapsids and SV_{40} virions in the same nucleus of a monkey cell, and figure 105 shows SV_5 nucleocapsids in the cytoplasm and SV_{40} virions in the nucleus of the same cell.

In general practice, latent virus infections in primary cell cultures are often *not recognized*. Viruses isolated from or virus stocks and virus vaccines made from such latently infected cultures would undoubtedly be contaminated with these endogenous agents. Precautions should therefore be taken whenever primary cell cultures, especially those derived from monkeys, are used. It is always advisable to use uninoculated control cultures in parallel for comparison.

VIRUSES OF NONPRIMATES

Latent virus infections are also found in the tissues, serum, or other animal products of a variety of nonprimate species. They include herpesvirus, from calf serum or in kidney tissues of guinea pigs, rabbits, rats, horses, dogs, and many other species; adenovirus from swine, bovine, and avian tissues; and small DNA viruses—the parvoviruses from rats and hamsters as well as papovaviruses from mice. Furthermore, certain viral agents have been recovered from animals previously considered germ-free. Thus one cannot be assured that the organs of any animal species are virus-free. These endogenous viruses have caused many problems for investigators in terms of interpreting results when an isolate is obtained from a clinical specimen.

Endogenous virus contaminants most commonly encountered in chicken embryo tissue culture are those that are egg-transmitted; these include avian lymphomatosis, avian encephalomyelitis, and Newcastle disease virus. Among these viruses, avian lymphomatosis is by far the most common and widespread. Avian encephalomyelitis virus and Newcastle disease virus may persist and are detectable in the choriollantoic fluids of infected embryos by various serologic methods.

The chicken embryo lethal orphan (CELO) virus, an adenovirus, is one of the more easily recognized endogenous contaminants of avian tissues. The virus, once activated, produces death in developing chicken embryos. If such an agent is recognized in avian tissues intended for cell culture, it is recommended that another source for embryonated eggs be found.

Table 30 lists some reported cases of virus isolation from cell cultures that

Table 30. Examples of Adventitious Viruses in Cell Cultures Prepared from Tissues of Domestic and Laboratory Animal and Avian Species

Animal Species	Virus Types
Domestic animals	
Cattle	adenovirus, herpesvirus, reovirus, parainfluenza virus, picornavirus
Horse	herpesvirus
Pig	adenovirus, picornavirus
Dog	adenovirus, herpesvirus, parainfluenza virus, reovirus
Laboratory animals	
Rabbit	poxvirus, papovavirus, herpesvirus
Guinea pig	herpesvirus, parainfluenza virus, retrovirus
Rat	parvovirus, herpesvirus, coronavirus
Hamster	parvovirus
Mouse	reovirus, papovavirus, leukovirus, coronavirus
Avian species	
Chicken	adenovirus, herpesvirus, myxovirus, leukovirus
Duck	herpesvirus, foamy-like virus

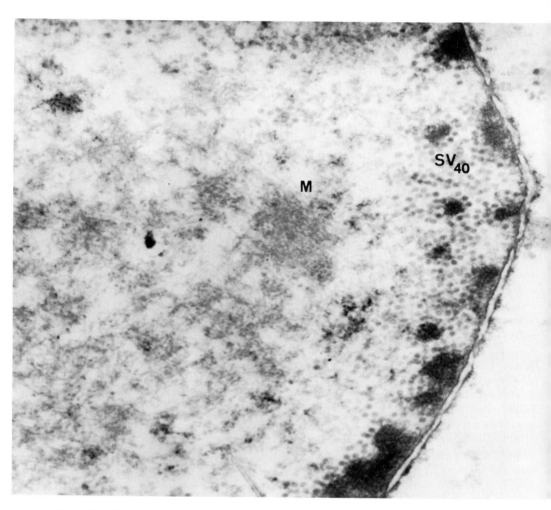

Figure 104. Electron micrograph showing mixed infection with measles virus and SV_{40} in a RhMK cell. A portion of a nucleus showing SV_{40} virions (SV_{40}) and measles virus (M) nucleocapsids (49,500X) (G. D. Hsiung et al., *Nature* (London) 215: 178, 1967).

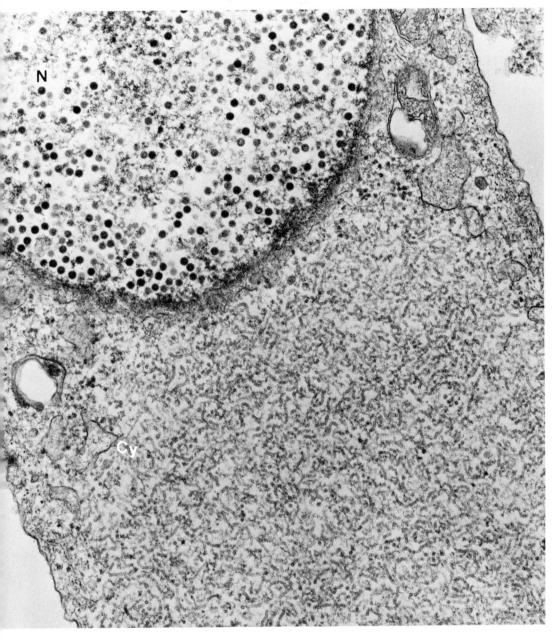

Figure 105. Electron micrograph showing a mixed infection with SV₅ and SV₄₀ in a GMK cell (C. K. Y. Fong and G. D. Hsiung, in *Virology and rickettsiology*, vol. 1, pt. 1, p. 104). SV₄₀ virions are showing in the nucleus (N) and SV₅ helical nucleocapsids in the cytoplasm (Cy) (48,000X).

were prepared from tissues of apparently healthy animals. These include both the DNA and RNA viruses; herpesviruses appear to be the most notorious. In addition, mycoplasmas have been found in certain mammalian and avian tissues although passaged cell lines are more often contaminated with these organisms. Any specimen or stock virus grown in these latently infected cultures is thus contaminated with an endogenous virus. Investigators should always keep in mind the possibility of the presence of an endogenous virus in the test system, especially when primary cell cultures are used. Methods for recognition of these viruses are similar to those described for the simian virus groups.

26. Culture Media, Reagents, and Solutions

The use of culture media in the propagation of mammalian cells has greatly expanded since Eagle's first report in 1955. The development and increased use of a large number of different primary and passaged cell cultures have resulted in an increased number of cell culture media that meet a variety of nutritional needs. Most if not all of the commonly used media may be obtained from commercial sources; some companies even provide custom service.

Sterile culture media may be purchased in a form ready for immediate use or for use after the addition of certain components. Many media may be purchased in concentrated form, usually 10X, so that reconstitution can be performed as needed. The latter offers advantages when storage is a problem. Powdered medium for tissue culture has been convenient for large laboratories, although it requires additional filtration equipment and further testing for sterility and cell growth. In certain instances, investigators prefer to prepare their own media and solutions. The few described below are simple and can be prepared with minimal laboratory facilities. Preference of antibiotics used in culture media varies from laboratory to laboratory. The amounts listed below for penicillin and streptomycin are given in parentheses to indicate that they should be added as needed. For additional information, see p. 270. All water used in the following formulas should be demineralized.

CULTURE MEDIA

Hanks' Balanced Salt Solution 10X

Solution A		*1 liter*	*5 liters*
	NaCl	80 gm	400 gm
	KCl	4 gm	20 gm
	$MgSO_4 \cdot 7H_2O$	1 gm	5 gm
	$MgCl_2 \cdot 6H_2O$	1 gm	5 gm
	$CaCl_2$ (anhydrous)	1.4 gm	7 gm
	Glucose	10 gm	50 gm
	Distilled water	800 ml	4000 ml
Solution B			
	$Na_2HPO_4 \cdot 2H_2O$	0.6 gm	3 gm
	KH_2PO_4	0.6 gm	3 gm
	Distilled water	200 ml	1000 ml

1. Weigh each salt in the order listed; dissolve in demineralized water.
2. Autoclave solutions A and B separately at 15 pounds for 15 minutes.
3. Mix A and B when cool; pour B into A *slowly*, stirring constantly.
4. Dispense in 100- to 500-ml amounts in sterile bottles and stopper tightly.
5. Store at room temperature or 4°C.

Hanks' Balanced Salt Solution 1X

	1 liter	*5 liters*
Distilled water, sterile	889.0 ml	4445.0 ml
Hanks' 10X	100.0 ml	500.0 ml
$NaHCO_3$ (7.5%)	7.0 ml	35.0 ml
Phenol red (0.5%)	4.0 ml	20.0 ml
Penicillin 200,000 units/ml	(1 ml)	(5 ml)
Streptomycin 500,000 µg/ml	(0.4 ml)	(2 ml)

Using sterile precautions:
1. Combine each solution in order listed above; final pH, 7.0–7.2.
2. Mix well and dispense in 500- to 1000-ml amounts.
3. Culture 1–5 ml in thioglycollate broth for sterility test.
4. Store in refrigerator.

Melnick's Medium A, Hanks' Growth Medium (HLS)
for Primary Monkey Kidney Cell Culture

	1 liter	*5 liters*
Distilled water, sterile	769 ml	3845 ml
Hanks' 10X	100 ml	500 ml
Lactalbumin hydrolysate (5%)	100 ml	500 ml
Calf serum (sterile)	20 ml	100 ml
NaHCO$_3$ (7.5%)	7 ml	35 ml
Phenol red (0.5%)	4 ml	20 ml
Penicillin, 200,000 units/ml	(1 ml)	(5 ml)
Streptomycin, 500,000 µg/ml	(0.4 ml)	(2 ml)

Using sterile precautions:
1. Add each solution in order listed above.
2. Mix well and dispense in 500- to 1000-ml amounts in sterile bottles; stopper lightly; final pH, 7.0–7.2.
3. Culture 1–5 ml in thioglycollate broth for sterility test.
4. Store in refrigerator.

Earle's Balanced Salt Solution 10X

Solution A

	1 liter	*5 liters*
NaCl	68 gm	340 gm
KCl	4 gm	20 gm
MgSO$_4$·7H$_2$O	2 gm	10 gm
NaH$_2$PO$_4$·H$_2$O	1.4 gm	7 gm
Glucose	10 gm	50 gm
Distilled water, sterile	800 ml	4000 ml

Solution B

CaCl$_2$ (anhydrous)	2 gm	10 gm
Distilled water, demineralized	200 ml	1000 ml

1. Dissolve each salt in demineralized water in the order listed above.
2. Autoclave solutions A and B separately at 15 pounds for 15 minutes.
3. Mix solutions A and B when cool; pour B into A; stir *slowly*.
4. Dispense in 100- to 500-ml amounts in sterile bottles and stopper tightly.
5. Culture 1–5 ml in thioglycollate broth for sterility test.
6. Store at room temperature or 4°C.

Melnick's Medium B, Earle's Maintenance Medium (ELS)
for Primary Monkey Kidney Cell Culture

	1 liter	*5 liters*
Distilled water, sterile	746 ml	3730 ml
Earle's 10X	100 ml	500 ml
Lactalbumin hydrolysate (5%)	100 ml	500 ml
Calf serum (sterile)	20 ml	100 ml
NaHCO$_3$ (7.5%)	30 ml	150 ml
Phenol red (0.5%)	4 ml	20 ml
Penicillin, 200,000 units/ml	(1 ml)	(5 ml)
Streptomycin, 500,000 µg/ml	(0.4 ml)	(2 ml)

Using sterile precautions:
1. Mix solutions in order listed above; final pH, 7.6–7.8.
2. Dispense in 500- to 1000-ml amounts.
3. Culture 1–5 ml in thioglycollate broth for sterility test.
4. Store in refrigerator.

Earle's Special Maintenance Medium (ES)
for Isolation of Myxovirus in Monkey Kidney Cell Culture

	1 liter	*5 liters*
Distilled water, sterile	867 ml	4335 ml
Earle's 10X	100 ml	500 ml
Bovine serum (fetal, ultrafiltrate)	20 ml	100 ml
NaHCO$_3$ (7.5%)	9 ml	45 ml
Phenol red (0.5%)	4 ml	20 ml
Penicillin, 200,000 units/ml	(1 ml)	(5 ml)
Streptomycin, 500,000 µg/ml	(0.4 ml)	(2 ml)

Using sterile precautions:
1. Mix solutions in order listed above; final pH, 6.8–7.0.
2. Distribute in 500- to 1000-ml amounts.
3. Culture 1–5 ml in thioglycollate broth for sterility test.
4. Store at 4°C.

Eagle's Basal Medium with 10% Calf Serum (EHS)

	1 liter	5 liters
Distilled water, sterile	765 ml	3825 ml
Hanks' 10X	100 ml	500 ml
Phenol red (0.5%)	4 ml	20 ml
Amino acids 100X*	10 ml	50 ml
NaOH (1N), adjusted to pH 7.0	(5 ml)	(25 ml)
Vitamins 100X*	10 ml	50 ml
Calf serum	100 ml	500 ml
$NaHCO_3$ (7.5%)	4.5 ml	23 ml
Penicillin, 200,000 units/ml	(1 ml)	(5 ml)
Streptomycin, 500,000 µg/ml	(0.4 ml)	(2 ml)
L-Glutamine stock solution (2.9%)†	10 ml	50 ml

*Purchased from a commercial source.
†L-Glutamine stock solution can be sterilized by filtration and stored at −20°C; add to the medium just before use.

Using sterile precautions:
1. Mix each solution in order listed; final pH 7.0–7.2.
2. Dispense in 500- to 1000-ml amounts.
3. Culture 1–5 ml in thioglycollate broth for sterility test.
4. Store at 4°C.

Eagle's Maintenance Medium with 5% Calf Serum (EES)

	1 liter	5 liters
Distilled water, sterile	790 ml	3950 ml
Earle's 10X	100 ml	500 ml
Phenol red (0.5%)	4 ml	20 ml
Amino acids 100X*	10 ml	50 ml
NaOH (1N), adjusted to pH 7.0	(5 ml)	(25 ml)
Vitamins 100X*	10 ml	50 ml
Calf serum	50 ml	250 ml
$NaHCO_3$ (7.5%)	29.6 ml	148 ml
Penicillin, 200,000 units/ml	(1 ml)	(5 ml)
Streptomycin, 500,000 µg/ml	(0.4 ml)	(2 ml)
L-Glutamine stock solution (2.9%)†	10 ml	50 ml

*Purchased from a commercial source.
†L-Glutamine stock solution can be sterilized by filtration and stored at −20°C; add to the medium just before use.

Using sterile precautions, follow the same procedures as for EHS. The final pH should be 7.6–7.8.

Lactalbumin Hydrolysate (5%)

Lactalbumin hydrolysate	50 gm
Distilled water	1000 ml

1. Weigh lactalbumin hydrolysate and dissolve in water using low heat (56°C water bath preferable).
2. Dispense in 100- to 200-ml amounts into bottles.
3. Autoclave at 10 pounds for 10 minutes.
4. Culture 1 ml into thioglycollate broth for sterility test.
5. Store in refrigerator or at room temperature.

REAGENTS AND SOLUTIONS

Phosphate-Buffered Saline (PBS)

Solution A

	1 liter	*5 liters*
NaCl	8.0 gm	40 gm
KCl	0.2 gm	1 gm
$CaCl_2 \cdot 2H_2O$	0.132 gm	0.66 gm
$MgCl_2 \cdot 6H_2O$	0.1 gm	0.5 gm
Distilled water	800 ml	4000 ml

Solution B

Na_2HPO_4	1.15 gm	5.75 gm
KH_2PO_4	0.2 gm	1 gm
Distilled water	200 ml	1000 ml

1. Dissolve each salt in demineralized water in order listed.
2. Autoclave solutions A and B separately at 15 pounds for 15 minutes.
3. Mix A and B when cool; pour B into A; *stir slowly*; final pH 7.0.
4. Dispense in 500- to 1000-ml amounts into sterile bottles.
5. Culture 1–5 ml in thioglycollate broth for sterility test.
6. Store in refrigerator.

Trypsin Solution in PBS 2.5%

PBS	1000 ml
Trypsin (1:300) (Difco)	25 gm

1. Add trypsin to PBS and shake to dissolve.
2. Filter through Seitz filter pad.
3. Dispense in 200- to 500-ml amounts into sterile bottles.
4. Culture 1–5 ml in thioglycollate broth for sterility test.
5. Store at −20°C.

Versene Solution (0.2%)

	1 liter	5 liters
NaCl	8 gm	40 gm
KCl	0.2 gm	1 gm
KH_2PO_4	0.2 gm	1 gm
Na_2HPO_4	1.15 gm	5.75 gm
Disodium ethylenediamine tetraacetate (EDTA)	0.2 gm	1 gm
Distilled water	1000 ml	5000 ml

1. Weigh each salt separately and dissolve in sequence.
2. Dispense in 50-ml amounts.
3. Autoclave at 15 pounds for 15 minutes.
4. Store at room temperature.

Trypsin-Versene Solution

Trypsin (2.5%)	5 ml
Versene (0.2%)	45 ml

1. Mix trypsin-versene using sterile procedures.
2. Before use, warm the mixture at 37°C in water bath.

Thioglycollate Broth for Bacteriological Sterility Tests

1. While stirring, add 24 gm thioglycollate (Difco) powder to 500 ml distilled water.
2. Add 5 gm dextrose.
3. Add sufficient distilled water to make 1 liter.
4. Dispense in 5-ml amounts into tubes.
5. Autoclave at 15 pounds for 15 minutes.
6. Store at room temperature in the dark.

$NaHCO_3$ (7.5%)

$NaHCO_3$	75 gm
Distilled water	1000 ml

1. Dissolve $NaHCO_3$ in sterile, demineralized water.
2. Filter through Seitz filter using *positive* pressure.
3. Dispense in 50- to 100-ml amounts into sterile bottles and stopper tightly.
4. Culture 1–5 ml in thioglycollate broth for sterility test.
5. Store in refrigerator or at room temperature.

Phenol Red (0.5%)

Phenol red	5 gm
NaOH (0.1N)	150 ml
Distilled water	850 ml

1. Add 0.1N NaOH to phenol red powder by drops until dissolved.
2. Add demineralized water.
3. Dispense in 100- to 500-ml amounts into bottles.
4. Autoclave at 15 pounds for 15 minutes.
5. Culture 1–2 ml into thioglycollate broth for sterility test.
6. Store at room temperature or in refrigerator, tightly stoppered.

Crystal Violet Solution for Cell Counts

Crystal violet	1 gm
Citric acid	19.2 gm
Distilled water	1000 ml

1. Dissolve citric acid in demineralized water.
2. Add crystal violet to above solution until it is dissolved.
3. Keep at room temperature.

Alsever's Solution

	1 liter
Dextrose	20.5 gm
Sodium citrate	8.0 gm
Citric acid	0.55 gm
NaCl	4.2 gm
Distilled water	1000 ml

1. Weigh each salt in the order listed above; dissolve in demineralized water.
2. Dispense in 50- to 100-ml amounts into bottles.
3. Autoclave at 10 pounds for 10 minutes.
4. Culture 1 ml into thioglycollate broth for sterility test.
5. Store stoppered solution at 4°C in refrigerator or at room temperature.

Antibiotic Stock Solutions

Name of Antibiotic	Stock Solution/ml	Final Concentration for Cultural Medium/ml	Treatment for Clinical Specimens/ml
Amphotericin B (Fungizone)	250 μg	1.25 μg	2.5 μg
Gentamicin	50,000 μg	50 μg	100 μg
Kanamycin	10,000 μg	50 μg	100 μg

Name of Antibiotic	Stock Solution/ml	Final Concentration for Cultural Medium/ml	Treatment for Clinical Specimens/ml
Neomycin	10,000 μg	50 μg	100 μg
Penicillin G	200,000 units	200 units	500 units
Streptomycin sulfate	500,000 μg	200 μg	500 μg
Tetracycline	10,000 μg	50 μg	100 μg

SUPPLEMENTARY READING FOR PART 4

Cell Culture Preparation

Book

Kruse, P. F., Jr., and Patterson, M. K., Jr., eds. *Tissue culture methods and applications*. New York: Academic Press, Inc., 1973.

Specific Articles

Bodian, D. Simplified method of dispersion of monkey kidney cells with trypsin. *Virology* 2: 575, 1956.

Youngner, J. S. Monolayer tissue cultures. I. Preparation and standardization of suspensions of trypsin-dispersed monkey kidney cells. *Proc. Soc. Exp. Biol. Med.* 85: 202, 1954.

Endogenous Contaminants in Cell Culture

Books and Review Papers

Barile, M. F. Mycoplasma contamination of cell cultures. In *Virology and rickettsiology*, ed. G. D. Hsiung and R. H. Green, vol. 1, pt. 2, p. 381. Handbook series in clinical laboratory science, Section H. West Palm Beach, Fla.: 1978.

Gillespie, J. H. Characteristics of cell culture systems. Viral flora of canine tissues. *Nat. Cancer Inst. Monogr.* 29: 133, 1968.

Hsiung, G. D. Latent virus infections in primate tissues with special reference to simian viruses. *Bact. Rev.* 32: 185, 1968.

Hsiung, G. D., Fong, C. K. Y., and Bia, F. Viruses of guinea pigs: considerations for biomedical research. *Micro. Rev.* 44: 468, 1980.

Hull, R. H. The simian viruses. Virol. Monogr. 2: 2, 1968.

Kelly, T. J., Jr., and Nathans, D. The genome of simian virus 40. *Adv. Virus Res.* 21: 85, 1977.

Kniazeff, A. J. Viruses infecting cattle and their role as endogenous contaminants of cell cultures. Cell culture for virus vaccine production. Nat. Cancer Inst. Monogr. 29: 123, 1968.

Melendez, L. V., and Daniel, M. D. Herpesvirus from South American monkeys. In *Medical primatology*, ed. E. J. Goldsmith and I. Moor-Jankowski, p. 686. Basel: Karger, 1971.

Malherbe, M. H. *Viral cytopathology*. Boca Raton, Fla.: CRC Press, Inc., 1980.

Smith, K. O. Adventitious viruses in cell cultures. *Prog. Med. Virol.* 12: 302, 1970.

Toolan, H. W. The picorna viruses. HRV and AAV. *Int. Rev. Exp. Path.* 6: 135, 1968.

Specific Articles

Chu, F. C., Johnson, J. B., Orr, H. C., Probst, P. G., and Petricciani, J. C. Bacterial virus contamination of fetal bovine sera. *In Vitro* 9: 81, 1973.

Croghan, D. L., Matchett, A., and Koski, T. A. Isolation of porcine parvovirus from commercial trypsin. *Appl. Microbiol.* 26: 431, 1973.

Hughes, J. H., and Hamparian, V. V. Commercial simian virus antiserum that inhibit virus replication in primary monkey kidney cell culture. *J. Clin. Micro.* 13: 824, 1981.

Lilynska, I., and Polna, I. Latent virus infection in primary monkey kidney cultures. *Acta Microbiol.* 5: 244, 1973.

Merrill, C. R., Friedman, T. B., Attallah, A. F. M., Geier, M. R., Krell, K., and Yarkin, R. Isolation of bacteriophages from commercial sera. *In Vitro* 8: 91, 1972.

Molander, C. W., Kniazeff, A. J., Boone, C. W., Paley, A., and Iwagawa, D. T. Isolation and characterization of viruses from fetal calf serum. *In Vitro* 7: 168, 1972.

Nettleton, P. F., and Rweyemamn, M. M. The association of calf serum with the contamination of BHK21 clone 12 suspension cells by a parvovirus serologically related to minute virus of mice (MVM). *Arch. Virol.* 64: 359, 1980.

Culture Media, Solutions, and Reagents

Review Papers

Swack, N. S. Cell cultures, culture media, reagents and endogenous viruses. In *Virology and rickettsiology*, ed. G. D. Hsiung and R. H. Green, vol. 1, pt. 2, p. 369. Handbook series in clinical laboratory science, Section H. West Palm Beach, Fla.: CRC Press, 1978.

Specific Articles

Eagle, H. Nutrition needs of mammalian cells in tissue culture. *Science* 122: 501, 1955.

Morton, H. I. A survey of commercially available tissue culture media. *In Vitro* 6: 89, 1970.

Rutzky, L. P., and Pumper, R. W. Supplement to a survey of commercially available tissue culture media (1970). *In Vitro* 9: 408, 1974.

Schafer, T. W., Pascale, A. Shimanaski, G., and Carne, P. E. Evaluation of gentamicin for use in virology and tissue culture. *Appl. Microbiol.* 23: 565, 1972.

Index